Dorothy

please return

A NURSE'S WAR

A
NURSE'S WAR

———◆———

Brenda McBryde

1979
CHATTO & WINDUS
LONDON

Published by
Chatto & Windus Ltd
40 William IV Street
London, WC2N 4DF

*

Clarke, Irwin & Co. Ltd
Toronto

British Library Cataloguing in Publication Data
McBryde, Brenda
    A nurse's war.
    1. McBryde, Brenda   2. Nurses – Biography
    I. Title
    610.73'092'4   RT37.M/
    ISBN 0–7011–2429–6

Set, printed and bound in Great Britain by
Cox & Wyman Ltd,
London, Fakenham and Reading

To the memory of
F. O. Helen M. Armstrong,
Women's Auxiliary Airforce

Acknowledgements

I wish to record my gratitude to Esther Corsellis for her constructive criticisms and to my husband for learning to cook.

Contents

Part I

Part II

Illustrations

Part I

1

The Royal Victoria Infirmary

It was not my lifelong ambition to become a nurse. I was not a dedicated Florence Nightingale from the cradle; nor was I following a hereditary profession. As far as I know, I was the only nurse in the family. But what do you do with a distinction in oral French, an addiction to diary keeping and an ability to draw? After two false starts in secretarial training and pharmacy I made a third, equally unsuitable, choice and as a first step towards independence, committed myself in the winter of 1938 to four years' training as a nurse at the Royal Victoria Infirmary, Newcastle-upon-Tyne. I was twenty years old. In the event, on thirty-six shillings a week and no salary at all for the first four months, my independence was questionable.

Newcastle was a grimy city in those days before smokeless fuel. Filth belched from its industrial chimneys, defiling its elegant seventeenth- and eighteenth-century buildings. The mediaeval tower of St. Nicholas' cathedral and the spires of another half-dozen ancient churches showed soot-black silhouettes against the northern sky. But the red-brick hospital set fair on the hill with the Town Moor at its back, had nothing to do with the dirt of the city. Solid and respectable it stood, its blank ward windows overlooking the figure of Queen Victoria set among beds of lobelia and alyssum. The nurses lived and studied in the adjoining Nurses' Home, insulated from disease and sickness by a dusty conservatory, and from the outside world by a strict regimen imposed by resident Home Sisters and Sister Tutors.

The Nurses' Home also housed the classrooms of the Pre-liminary Training School where, to novices like myself, a six-week course of instruction was given before nursing started in earnest in the hospital. I remember the cramped wooden desks and waxed floor, the walls hung with illustrations of the human body, and on a raised dais at one end of the classroom Jimmie the skeleton and the Sister Tutor.

Twenty of us, uniformed in striped frocks, starched caps and aprons, black stockings and flat, lace-up shoes, were bent over notebooks. Our arms, bare to the elbow (we were not permitted to wear a cardigan), were goose-pimpled with cold. It was November. The immaculate Sister Tutor fired her dictation notes at such a rate that none of us could pause for an instant even to blow our noses as we scribbled page after page. I could hear boys kicking a football about on the frosty Town Moor near by, and lifting my head for a moment I glimpsed a butchers' lad through the window, whistling as he took a short cut around the back of the hospital, his bicycle tray full of black puddings. He inhabited a different world and one that grew increasingly attractive as the disciplines of a nurse's training began to bite.

We had to tread carefully through a maze of rules and some days we could do nothing right. One did not speak to a Tutor unless spoken to. No questions at all were permitted at lectures. When I had the temerity to correct an obvious grammatical mistake as I copied the Sister Tutor's notes into my lecture book, my punishment was to re-write the whole lecture – including the error.

Now, in bleak November, we were half-way through the course, our minds reeling with an extraordinary diversity of facts. We had learned the life-cycle of the bed-bug. We knew how to apply a leech and a tourniquet, and all about the ventilation system of the Houses of Parliament. We could make a bed and give an enema, take a pulse and measure medicine. We had been shown how to bath, bandage, poultice, purge, comb for nits and reverently carry out Last Offices on a pink and white life-size dummy.

The lecture today was on anatomy and we were writing down strange, euphonious words like 'internal saphenous' and 'haemolyticus streptococcus' and 'the Isles of Langerhans'. It sounded splendid but incomprehensible to me. I had a terrible cough and was finding concentration difficult. At my original interview with the Matron of the hospital I had mentioned that

I had been nursing my little nephew who had whooping cough, but the fact had passed without comment. Now my bouts of coughing were disrupting the lecture.

'The one with the cough,' the Sister Tutor enunciated crisply. 'Stand outside.'

I coughed my way into the corridor and closed the classroom door behind me, feeling sick. I want to go to bed I told myself in deep self-pity, and reflected that now I would have to borrow someone else's notes in order to complete the anatomy lecture.

The chink of keys and the flat pad-pad of sensible shoes announced the approach of the Home Sister. Bulky, black-uniformed, wearing her habitual face of disapproval, she trundled around the corner and found me sagging against the wall.

'What are you doing here, Nurse?'

Wearily, I explained.

'Stand up straight, then. Tuck in your hair, and remember to address me as "Sister".' And she swung ponderously off down the passage to look for cigarette ends in the lavatory.

The following day, I was instructed by the Home Sister to report sick, and the medical Registrar whose duties included care of the nursing staff made the predictable diagnosis of whooping cough. I was less popular than ever with the authorities. 'Bringing her germs here . . .'

Dressed once more in civilian clothes, I sat in my bedroom awaiting the ambulance that was to take me to Walkergate Isolation Hospital, already an outcast behind a sheet soaked in disinfectant that hung from my door. I sat as still as stone on my high, hard bed, my back against the wall, trying to keep at bay the hovering paroxysm of coughing. Without a preliminary knock, the door was pushed open and the Home Sister came in, knocking her cap askew against the sheet and showing wispy, white hair. She was old and should have been dozing in a rocking chair with a cat.

'Here,' she said gruffly. I think she had forgotten how to speak with gentleness. From a deep pocket as big as a pillowslip she fished out an orange. 'Put this in your case and don't start feeling sorry for yourself. The ambulance is waiting.'

I followed her along the passage, lugging my case behind me, glad to be leaving this uncharitable place. There, I told myself, goes my one and only attempt to become a nurse.

That is what I thought in the blue light of the ambulance in the winter of 1938, but at the Isolation Hospital I discovered, as a patient, what nursing is all about. With a high fever, I learned the relief that tepid sponging can bring to burning limbs, and the difference between a gentle touch and a too-hearty grasp on sensitive skin. I came to appreciate the comfort of a cool, correctly placed pillow, of sheets without creases to lie on, and how carelessly handled crockery can sound like a clap of thunder to a throbbing head. I knew the frustration of the empty water jug, and requests made twice but not repeated for fear of being thought a nuisance. Most of all, I came to know the blessed contentment that a patient experiences when the good nurse is on duty. I discovered then that I wanted to be a nurse.

January 1939 saw me back in Newcastle at the Royal Victoria Infirmary, starting all over again. After the Training School, four years of practical work on the wards faced me, and two state examinations, the Preliminary and the Final, with an internal hospital examination somewhere between. At the end I would be able to write S.R.N. (State Registered Nurse) after my name.

Back I went with twenty fresh recruits, back to the same irksome disciplines, but this time with a difference. I had grown extra defences during my convalescence and this time the rebuffs bounced straight off. I found everything in the curriculum of interest and therefore not difficult to memorise. The class passed uneventfully from the Training School to the wards and within six weeks I was a real nurse.

The hospital was a kingdom on its own, a carefully graded society of doctors, nurses and domestics, held in a framework of unwritten laws. Consultant surgeons and physicians, as heads of the medical 'firms', dispensed their variable humours along with clinical instruction to the medical students. The Ward

Sister's authority over patients and nurses alike was immense, but an uneasy alliance existed between herself and the ward-maid whose years of service frequently exceeded her own. The ward-maid polished the floors just so long as no questions were asked about her other activities. When she left for home each night, there was often more than her working shoes in the ward-maid's shopping basket. Choice pieces of patients' chicken (filched from the ward larder) would sometimes find their way wrapped in a copy of the *Daily Worker*, but it would be a brave nurse who dared denounce her. At the bottom of the pecking order came the junior probationer nurse who was fair game for everyone from the ward-maid upwards.

The identical, white-tiled wards were full of miners and factory workers, folk to be dosed and douched, investigated and operated upon, and sometimes sent home to die when the right answers were not to be found in the medical books of 1939. In the Out-Patients' Department, time stood still. Men and women with blank faces sat on wooden benches there, waiting for medical attention and clutching appointment cards. Many sick people spent the greater part of a day awaiting their turn, their only diversion being the traffic of casualties coming in from the town, the boilermaker with a cut tendon, the housewife wheezing with asthma, the little boy with his head stuck in a chamber pot.

To the casual passer-by walking his dog in the Leazes, this was the Royal Victoria Infirmary, a fine hospital that one might be grateful for one day. The brick walls gave no hint of the unreal world within where no sounds intruded of the town below. The sea-gulls by the fish-quay and the clanging trams were all far away from this aseptic, rubber-soled institution. When summer came, it was not allowed to cross the threshold and all the fragrances of sea salt and fresh grass cuttings and heavy-headed roses were overwhelmed at once in disinfectant. This place of polished floors and Victorian curlicues, of geometric counterpanes and infinite cleanliness was where I lived and worked.

At the beginning of August, only weeks away from the crisis

that was about to break over Europe, I had six months' experience under my belt. I was junior probationer on Mens' Surgical Ward 4. Alternately bewildered by awful responsibilities on the one hand, and the denial of any adult freedom on the other, I had somehow come through that testing six months. There had been sleepless nights over the man whose urine I had forgotten to measure.

'If he dies, it will be because of your negligence,' the Ward Sister had said in the hearing of the patients. I was rarely out of trouble. I could not get my counterpane corners angled correctly and once I was caught accepting a 'black bullet' (locally produced peppermints) from a miner. The hours were cruelly long, sixty-seven hours a week, and we junior nurses found that our aching feet swelled like pumpkins. Yet, in spite of the day-to-day miseries, most of us were very keen and very willing. As the weeks went by, mistakes became less frequent, or else we learned to hide them. My feet hardened up with a nightly application of methylated spirit and talcum powder. I was determined to survive.

Some did not. Four of the twenty girls in my training set gave up to go back to Mum or take up hairdressing. The rest of us soldiered on, getting our reward from the patients themselves (they were always on our side), and from a growing fascination with the work. The circulation of the blood was a revelation, and the kidney a miracle of engineering. Occasionally there were moments when a grateful relative could make one feel six feet tall, not a cloth-headed junior any more.

Now, one August evening, I was in the ward sluice, rinsing out the last of the urinals and tidying up the sink. There had been a pit disaster that day at one of the many collieries near Newcastle and ten injured miners had been admitted to Ward 4, white eyes red-rimmed in black faces. I spent most of the afternoon washing the coal dust from their bodies and my apron was streaked with dirt. I looked as though I had been down a mine myself. One by one, the injured men were taken to the operating theatre and the Staff Nurse and myself, the only two nurses on duty that afternoon, had to work fast to get them cleaned up in time and to prepare beds for their return. With the Sister out of the way, I was no longer scared and I glowed with pride when my Staff Nurse said 'Thanks, Mac'.

The clock at the entrance to the ward said five minutes to six. Five minutes to go. I had been on duty since seven o'clock that morning and my legs ached. Peter Aynsley was calling for me that evening. We would go somewhere. It did not matter where as long as something to eat was provided. The food in the hospital was poor and there was never enough of it.

Six o'clock. I knocked on the door of the Ward Sister's office. Yes, I had cleaned the sluice and collected the specimens. Yes, I had made the barley water and emptied Number Two's Winchester bottle.

In the corridor ahead of me was Edna Bramley. At twenty-three, Edna was a little older than the average student and had given up a lucrative secretarial position in order to train as a nurse. We all thought she should have her head examined. I hurried to catch up with her. Must not run. Only in cases of fire or haemorrhage is a nurse permitted to run. The corridor was filling up with nurses going off duty and there would be a rush for baths. We hurried past the main operating theatre and the Children's Ward where babies bawled indignantly. We joined the stream of nurses filing through the conservatory, probationers' striped frocks giving way to Staff Nurse blue and everyone to the mauve of a Ward Sister. To break precedence was almost a bread-and-water charge. Even the six-week seniority between one Training School and the next was most jealously guarded.

Returning to my room after my bath, I found Jean Williams, one of my training set, sitting on my bed, wrapped in a jazzy, silk dressing gown, looking miserable.

'What's up with you?'

'I'm going on Nights tonight.'

I closed the door. Our first spell of night-duty was overdue and we had been expecting it. Now Jean was the first of the crowd to go. She looked terribly vulnerable, sitting there with her spaniel eyes.

'It would have to be me.'

I began dressing. Peter would be here in a few minutes, but I knew how she must feel. She was so nervous that she had not been able to sleep at all during the day. She would be half-dead by the morning. At that moment, a car horn sounded beneath my window and Peter was there in his old Morris.

Everyone at the Black Bull was talking about the Polish crisis and Peter was working himself up into a fine state of excitement. 'The Territorials will be called up first thing,' he assured me with satisfaction as we sat down to plates of ham and eggs and pickled onions. He had enlisted during the Czech crisis of the previous year. 'Anything's better than the office.'

With all the talk of war in the pub, Peter and I did not notice the time flying by and it was twenty minutes past ten when we arrived back at the hospital gates. I was twenty minutes late. If my name was taken by the porter at the gate, I would be for the Matron's office in the morning and one of my two precious monthly late passes would be forfeited. So I decided to go over the railings at a point where shrubbery inside the grounds broke the fall. With a little help from Peter, I was over the top and on my way.

As I struggled out of the sooty rhododendrons, the half-hour chimes sounded from St. Thomas' in the Haymarket. Half past ten. 'Lights Out' in the Nurses' Home. The Night Super would be starting her rounds of the hospital.

I made for the gynaecological ward which adjoined the conservatory leading to the Nurses' Home. Much depended on who was on duty there as to how much co-operation there would be. I climbed the fire escape at the rear of the ward and noted the fact that lights were still on inside. A bad sign. Most of the other wards were in darkness by now. The gynaecological ward must be busy. I crossed the balcony and tried the double glass doors but, predictably, they were locked, and my fears were confirmed as I peered inside.

There was a theatre trolley at the other end under a blaze of lights. Red screens and relatives were around the bedside of one seriously ill woman, and night lights glimmered over blood transfusions at three other beds. No doubt about it, I would be pretty unpopular with whoever was in charge here tonight.

The junior nurse emerged from the red screens at that moment and I tapped loudly on the window pane to attract her attention. To my immense relief, I saw it was Jean Williams. She did not hear my knocking but a patient near the doors did and called out. Jean came hurrying down. I saw her turn towards the balcony with a look of annoyance which lessened only slightly when she saw it was me. She glared with some hostility as she opened the door.

'Where on earth have you been?' she demanded. 'Look at your frock and your face is all black.'

'Has the Night Super been yet?' This was no time for explanations.

'She's been on and off the ward all evening. We've had four admissions, all for the theatre, and now you.'

I was starting to walk up the ward beside her when my heart turned over. The Night Super was breezing down the corridor into the ward at that very moment, followed by a porter pushing a lumpy figure on a trolley. I flung myself face-down over the polished floor and slid like a puck over ice under the nearest bed, praying that the darkness at this end of the ward would conceal me. Jean seemed to have taken root where she stood. Her eyes filled with fright as they followed the progress of the Night Super and she seemed quite unable to move. This was a clear case of 'Night Nurse's Paralysis', a strange syndrome common amongst night nurses when caught breaking the rules. In an emergency, the brain's message for action does not get through. It is something to do with lack of sleep. Jean was not snapping out of it and I could see the Night Super on her way down to our end of the ward.

Under the bed, I hardly dared to breathe as swishing skirt noises brought sturdy shoes within my vision.

'Anything wrong, Nurse?'

I willed Jean to speak but it was the patient in the bed above me who came to the rescue.

'Only me, Sister. I was just asking for a bedpan.'

The feet shifted and took up their 45° stance not twelve inches from my nose. I heard Jean rush off to the sluice.

'Are you feeling better, Mrs. Fairbairn?'

It was said that Sister Paton, the Night Super, knew the name of every patient in the hospital. This much-respected woman had chosen permanent night-duty so that she could look after her invalid father during the day. By night, the responsibility for the hospital was hers alone.

The feet moved away and I heard the trolley creaking as the porter took the case to the theatre. The lights went out at the top of the ward and I crawled cautiously from under the bed. The woman lying there, so thin she barely made a bump under the counterpane, smiled at me, a skin-tight smile on a face ravaged by septicaemia.

'Thanks,' I whispered. 'You saved my bacon.'

'That's aa'reet,' she sighed wearily. 'Why shouldn't you bits of lasses have some fun.'

I was on night-duty myself by the end of the week and had to cancel a date with Peter. As it happened, he would not have been able to make it anyhow. All Territorials had been re-quested to report to their nearest barracks and he had a drill practice that night.

The Polish problem was no nearer a solution. We pored over the patients' newspapers. Rumours thrived. We were to be a military hospital. All patients were to be evacuated. But every-thing was normal on my first shift of night-duty. I hurried on to Ward 5 at nine o'clock in the evening, my lecture books under my arm and a screw of tea in my pocket.

It was Saturday night and Ward 5 was on Reception. I hur-ried non-stop from sluice to kitchen, secretion room to laundry, with wash-bowls, sputum mugs and armfuls of theatre clothing. Two duodenal ulcers perforated during the night and were brought in rigid with pain. A young man dived into an empty swimming pool after a party and cracked his skull. Two drunks, stinking of vomit, punched the living daylights out of each other and were cleaned up and sent to the theatre.

At midnight, I went to the first dinner sitting and carried my plate of grey, boiled beef to a suitably unpresumptuous seat at the bottom of the table beside Edna and Jean. The stale smell of the dining-room was more pronounced at night; it was a smell compounded from years of boiled cabbage and synthetic lemon jelly piquantly spiked with disinfectant. The tea brewing and the meat stewing on the hotplate made the green-painted walls weep with moisture. Naked electric light bulbs did nothing to conceal the unloveliness of the place where we took our refreshment.

Jean gave me a nod. She was now quite accustomed to night-duty and had the advantage of me. 'Where are you?'

'Five. We're on Reception.'

'Busy?'

'Like Paddy's Fair. Drunks, the lot.'

'For God's sake cut out the shop.' The withering comment came from a nurse sitting six months further up the table and the three of us relapsed into silence.

There were only two nurses to a ward on night-duty so when my senior nurse went to dinner I was left in charge. She handed me the keys to the dangerous drugs cupboard, picked up her magazine and patted her pocket for cigarettes. 'Watch the intravenous drips. Keep a close eye on the ops. for haemorrhage and give Bed 3's relatives a cup of tea.'

I tried to keep an intelligent look on my face and quell the beginnings of panic in my breast. For the next forty-five minutes, I was in charge of a ward full of men, some of whom were very ill. I pinned the keys to the inside of my pocket and prayed that no-one would die. I tip-toed right around the ward, peering at each patient to make sure he was breathing.

'Boo!' said the footballer with the cartilage and I nearly jumped out of my skin.

I made tea for Bed 3's relatives, perched, sleepless on their chairs behind the red screens, counting the puff-puff breaths of the pale young man in bed. I checked the drips and looked at the theatre dressings. Then one of the two drunks began to emerge from anaesthesia. Sitting bolt upright in bed, his bandaged head bloody but unbowed, he began to recite the twenty-third psalm at the top of his voice, wakening the whole ward.

'The Lor-r-d is my Shepherd,

He maketh me to lie down. . .'

'Gan on, then,' said a cross old man in the next bed. 'Lie doon and be done wi' it.'

'I wish He'd make ye shut yer gob,' sighed the footballer with resignation.

Back from dinner, my senior roughed in her night report, leaving a space alongside Bed 3, and I went to test urines in the secretion room. Four o'clock is the dead hour for those on night-duty. This dank, still period just before the dawn, when the spirit is at its lowest, is entirely alien. Three o'clock still carries with it sympathetic vestiges of the night before, but four o'clock is on another waveband altogether. For the nurse on night-duty this gap of time, before the birds wake and the sky lightens, has nothing to commend it. Her second wind has not yet arrived and her only sensations are of goose pimples, desolation and utter fatigue.

It was just before four o'clock when the hesitant breathing behind the screens tailed away in a tiny hiccough. Gauche and inadequate, I hurried to fetch my senior who, at twenty-two, was all at once mature and wise, able to give comfort and strength to the bereaved. They wandered away, mouselike and heartbroken, through the echoing corridors, trying to comprehend their loss as they made for the first tram home. I went for my half-hour tea break.

'On your way back, bring a shroud from the linen room.' My senior removed the pillow from under the young man's head.

In the soupy dining-room, I pushed aside my plate and cup, laid my head on the table and slept for ten blissful minutes with my hair in the jam.

Within a few days, there was only one subject on everybody's mind, one topic of conversation. Would there be war? Parliament had been recalled from summer recess. We began to realise that the Polish crisis, unlike the Czech crisis of the previous year, was not going away. Gas masks were distributed to civilians and half-finished air-raid shelters were hastily completed. The Town Moor was ripped across with trenches and stuck with concrete teeth to prevent it being used as an enemy landing ground. Children were evacuated to the safety of the countryside.

On 27th August, evacuation from the hospital of all but the very seriously ill patients began. Plump ladies with gallbladders, their drainage bottles precariously strapped to their sides, were jollied on to stretchers and into the waiting ambulances. Old men with tubes, orthopaedic patients rigid in plaster of Paris, all had to be wrapped in blankets and transported with their baccy and their gas-masks, knitting and false teeth, to the cottage hospitals and convalescent homes of the peaceful Northumbrian countryside.

'What aboot me pension, Norse?'

'How's me dowter ganna find us?'

'The paper lad owes us a tanner.'

That night I went on to a strangely changed ward. The light bulbs had been painted blue and what little illumination they cast was weird and depressing. Every vestige of daylight from ground floor windows was blotted out by walls of sandbags. Army trucks had been delivering them to the hospital all day. The few remaining patients were edgy all night, wanting drinks, cough mixtures and bottles. No-one slept very much.

The third of September was Edna Bramley's birthday. It was a fine Sunday morning and we were getting ready for bed. Church bells were ringing for the morning service and house wives were beating the batter for Yorkshire pudding.

'My father will probably have to go,' said Edna, grave at the thought. All holiday leave in the hospital had been cancelled. The Territorials were on stand-by.

'What about us?' I wondered.

'No good till we're State Registered.'

'It'll be over by then,' I said with disgust.

'It hasn't started yet.'

But that night, the lights were out all over the land and cars nudged dangerously along unlit roads with only a pinprick of light showing through masked headlights. At my home in Whitley Bay, fat coils of barbed wire snaked across the deserted sands and anti-tank traps appeared as fast as the concrete could set.

We were at war.

2

At War

Once the Prime Minister had made his announcement that we were at war, it was like turning a corner and looking at familiar objects from a new angle. Institutions of great permanence now seemed curiously expendable. People leading humdrum lives found that doors were opening for them, that change was in the air.

Unwary holidaymakers caught on the wrong side of the Channel rushed to get seats on the last ferries leaving the Hook, Calais and Boulogne as though German tanks were already crossing the Rhine. Peter, an insurance clerk no more, took up residence in the Gateshead Drill Hall and was given two stripes and a manual on gun maintenance.

Barrage balloons like fat silver fishes rose giddily over the shipyards on the Tyne, their tethering cables set to ensnare the expected hordes of low-flying enemy aircraft. The hospital, empty of patients for the first time in its history, waited.

After we had scrubbed and polished the lockers and cupboards, and spring-cleaned the sluices and bathrooms, we set to making dressings. Mountains of gauze, lint and cotton wool were demolished in the making of wound dressings, swabs, eye pads and many-tailed bandages. We padded a forest of splints and sewed a depressing supply of shrouds. A Nissen hut to be known as a Decontamination Centre was set up in the hospital grounds, equipped with resuscitation apparatus and army folding beds. None of us was allowed to stir a foot outside the hospital without a gas-mask and the special identity cards which entitled us to priority transport back to hospital in the event of an air raid. But the anticipated bombardment did not come. The September sky remained serenely empty of raiding bombers.

A strange new freedom emerged on night-duty following the

declaration of war. Sitting under the blue lights of the empty ward, busy with scissors, gauze and cotton wool, I came to know my senior nurse, Anne Newsome, better than would have been possible in normal times. She was a very attractive girl with a confident manner that was as good as a transfusion to a nervous patient.

Medical students appeared from nowhere as soon as the Night Super had finished her rounds. Russell Slater was one of the regulars. He was on standby duty for air raids one night when he paid us a visit, happily timed to coincide with our illicit brew-up at about eleven o'clock.

'I've got news for you,' he said. 'We're opening for civvie patients again at the end of the week. The Chief's getting worried. Too much surgery piling up.'

In a week, the hospital was back to normal except for two specified emergency wards. Some of the blue paint was scratched from light bulbs, and the sandbags, which were found to be harbouring fleas, were removed from all windows but those of the air raid wards.

Then on 17th October, we had the first air raid warning. Our blood froze to the banshee wailing of the sirens. Our instructions were to place each patient underneath his bed, wrapped in a blanket and with his gas mask to hand. In the urgency of the whooping siren, Anne Newsome and I looked down the dim ward at thirty-five anxious faces. Since most of the men were unable to get out of bed unaided, we were faced with a formidable task. The arrival of Russell Slater and another medical student, Ray Dobson, white coats over their pyjamas, was providential. We set about wrapping, lifting and reassuring the patients, some of whom had not the slightest idea of what was going on.

'Is the zeppelins coming, Norse?'

The floor was hard on their old bones and some of their drainage apparatus developed hydraulic difficulties like airlocks and flood-backs. We were all four of us exhausted by the time our instructions had been carried out and thirty-five pairs of calloused feet stuck out from under the beds. Matron, hurriedly dressed, did an unheard-of night round of the hospital. Then the All Clear sounded and the whole operation went into reverse.

We did not know it then, but the planes were no nearer than the north coast of Scotland. The Luftwaffe might have been about to land on the Town Moor, so frantic was the activity in the hospital. Of the attacking planes, two were shot down into the sea where their pilots drifted for two days before being picked up near Whitby and interned.

After that, there was some fresh thinking about air raid procedure, and it was decided that the patients would be better left in their beds since very little protection was afforded by lying underneath, and the upheaval did most of them more harm than good. In future, our job was to check gas masks and convince the patients that bombs would not fall on the hospital.

There were no more excitements for a while. The First British Expeditionary Force was dug in on France's northern border. Uniformed men and women became commonplace on Newcastle's streets. My art student friend, Helen Armstrong, had volunteered, like Peter, during the Czech crisis, and now found herself posted as a member of the Women's Auxilliary Air Force to be assistant cook at the balloon barrage station at Benton. Peter collected another stripe.

'They're such a crumby lot,' he explained modestly. 'I'm brilliant by comparison.'

He had just been on an intensive training course and arranged to meet me one October afternoon when I should have been in bed. Nurses on night-duty were not allowed to get up before five p.m. but I set my alarm for three o'clock this day and, keeping a lively eye open for lurking Home Sisters, I nipped quickly through the hospital and down to the town. He was waiting for me in a dreary café that smelt of fried air. He told me that he expected embarkation leave any day now before joining the Expeditionary Force in France and I was mean with envy. One could not help feeling a certain excitement about the war. There was a longing to get into the action. But with less than one year's nursing training, my future seemed to be accounted for at the Royal Victoria Infirmary. It would be 1943 before I qualified.

Night-duty was supposed to stretch over twelve weeks but Edna Bramley and I had done fourteen before we went back on to day duty. With only two nights off a month, this had been a long, wearying stint, and towards the end of it, we felt continually tired.

We were becoming aware that, compared with other hospitals in the country, we worked longer hours for less pay. In some training hospitals, there was now a forty-eight hour working week while we were still relentlessly held to sixty-seven. We were grossly overworked, underfed and underpaid, but nurses of our year were too junior to make our complaints heard and, for the most part, too tired to protest.

On day duty, Edna was sent to a Women's Medical Ward where, to her gratification, she was able to recognise symptoms of the diseases we had been studying in theory; heart disease, asthma, anaemia, arterio-sclerosis.

I was sent as back-shop nurse to the main operating theatre. The back-shop of a theatre is like the scullery of a five star hotel. Everything goes in dirty and must come out clean, but in the back-shop, clean means sterile and dirty means bloody. I was filled with misgivings as I presented myself for duty that first morning. Timidly, I pushed open the double doors and went inside, to be halted at once by the noise: the clatter of enamel basins, the shriek of steam as it whistled through autoclaves, the bustle of scrubbing. The theatres were being cleaned. Through an open door, I could see a great overhead lamp blazing down on a tiled floor running with soap suds. An unseen hand sent enamel bowls spinning over the wet floor and an operating table glided by. Jets of water played down the tiled walls and gurgled along the drains. As I hesitated, a wet towel whizzed out of a dark aperture next to the theatre and landed at my feet, quickly followed by others. Moving in the direction from which they came, I found a figure in white Wellington boots bending over a sink in a small room full of steam. She was sluicing stained linen and hurling it over her shoulder to join the pile outside as if her life depended on it. I cupped my hands and shouted against the noise of hissing steam and bubbling sterilisers.

'I'm the new back-shop.'

She turned. Her fair skin was flushed with the steam and damp strands of ginger hair escaped from a square of linen tied closely over her head. A look of delight spread over her face. 'Thank God for that!' she shouted above the din. 'Staff Nurse is in the anaesthetic room. Go and report.'

The Staff Nurse took her eyes away from the instruments she was laying out for only an instant. 'Tell Alderton she takes over from Proctor.'

'Alderton?'

'Back-shop. She'll tell you what to do. Get changed and be quick about it. The list starts at nine-thirty.'

There were no boots my size and the only gown left would have fitted an elephant. I clomped over to claim the back-shop and Alderton, now promoted, gabbled off a string of instructions before disappearing in a flurry of importance through the theatre door. She was a tall girl, with eyelashes like sawdust over pale, resentful eyes.

'You're not allowed to put a foot inside here,' she said imperiously. 'I'll bring you the dirty instruments at the end of every case.'

I nodded. Back-shop nurse was the lowest form of life.

'Scrub them and bung 'em back in the steriliser double quick. It's Piggy Trotter and he's murder.'

None of this encouraged my already shaky spirit. I looked about me. The whole place resembled a devil's kitchen. An autoclave of gloves kept going off like a pressure cooker and cylinders of boiling water rumbled and rattled as if they might explode at any moment.

'Sterile airways!' bawled the Staff Nurse from the anaesthetic room.

'Lotions!' shouted Alderton from the theatre.

A porter wandered up to me, scratching his head. 'Where's your chit? Can't take your laundry without a chit.'

Somehow, by nine o'clock, the scrubbing and the clattering

had ceased. Trolleys in the theatre were set with sterile instruments; hand-bowls in stands were filled with antiseptic lotions; the Staff Nurse was scrubbed up and ready. The Sister in charge hovered nervously, checking the time, the dressings, the sutures. The uneasy silence was suddenly shattered by the dramatic arrival of the surgeon who was operating that day.

Striding at the head of a procession of anxious medical students, he crashed back the double entrance doors, proclaiming his arrival in tones of such feudal arrogance that I unwisely left my refuge to investigate. A trolley, left in the passage by some unforgivable oversight on the part of a porter, projected into the Great Man's path. He thrust it angrily away from him as I emerged from my back-shop and I collected it square in my middle. Winded, and in agony, I let out a yell that stopped them all in their tracks. The surgeon turned and stared. All the students stared, numb with apprehension. To have 'the Chief' upset at the beginning of an operating list spelt disaster for everyone. The Sister's face went puce with annoyance.

'How dare you!' she snapped at me and led the greatly affronted surgeon to the changing room where his boots and little hat and special white trousers were laid out ready for him, all marked 'Mr. Trotter Only'.

'She's new, sir,' I heard her say.

'She's mad,' he growled. 'Keep her out of my way.'

Back at the sink, I swore darkly that if my spleen was ruptured, as it well might be, I would not allow that man to get within striking distance of me with a scalpel. I think I upset his day. Certainly nothing seemed to be going right in the theatre. I waited behind the closed door, holding my breath, and listened in alarm to the long silences punctuated by roars of rage and the tinkling of instruments on the floor. After every such instance, Alderton appeared at the door, eyes big with fright over the top of her mask.

'Quick!' She would thrust a handful of instruments into my hands. 'Sterilise these again.'

Self-defeating exercise, this, I thought as they went back into the theatre ready to be hurled away at the next bout of temper. I was thankful that I was only the back-shop nurse.

Then came my encounter with the leg. Nobody had warned me about that. Alderton appeared once more at the theatre door but this time, it was not a handful of instruments or a lotion jug she passed to me, but a leg, wrapped in a sterile towel, bristling with artery forceps. It was in my arms before I realised. The theatre door closed again and I was alone with it.

For one mad moment, I nearly took to my heels. I would run away – go and work in an armament factory, plant turnips with the Land Army – anything but deal with this monstrous bundle. Then I took a grip on myself. Hundreds of nurses must have done this before me, and if they could do it, so could I. I removed the artery forceps, scrubbed them and dropped them into the steriliser; removed the towels and sluiced them, then I took a firm grip on the leg and carried it off in search of a rubbish bin. There was nothing large enough in the theatre so I went off down the corridor to the nearest ward. Startled visitors with their bunches of flowers were no more upset than I was myself. Ward 7's bin, in a bay off the ward entrance, was the nearest but the leg did not fit, quite, and I had to balance the lid on the five yellow toes. I pulled in my stomach muscles very hard and returned to the theatre, feeling very pleased with myself.

This satisfaction did not last long. When the owner of the leg had been duly dispatched back to his bed, the door from the theatre into my back-shop opened and my friend, the surgeon, stood there, filling the doorway. He was addressing the students over his shoulder as he advanced. His eyes, travelling over the benches and the floor, flinched a little when they encountered me. I retreated, hands behind my back, until I felt the hot copper of the boiler. What on earth was he after now?

He pulled the mask down from his nose, a red nose, open-pored with the heat, and bent his brow to me, pressed against the boiler. 'Where is it?' he snapped.

I stuck out my chin and tried to appear casual. 'Where's what?'

'Where's the leg, Nurse?' screeched the Sister from the fringe of the crowd in my back-shop. 'Where have you put the leg?'

I was beginning to feel out of my depth. 'In Ward 7's rubbish bin,' I said and waited for the silence to break. There were little gasps from the students. It appeared that they were usually given instruction on dissection in cases like this.

'Then go and get it back again!' The Sister's voice had a tremble in it and was at least two tones higher. Muffled explosions kept going off among the medical students, some of whom were finding it difficult to keep a straight face, but my face was straight enough as I stalked back along the corridor.

The surgeon got his leg. He received it silently, regarding me with some curiosity, as if he thought I should be somewhere else, in a mental institution perhaps. I met his gaze with equal antagonism, holding hard on to what little dignity was left me. Five foot tall, wrapped in a six foot gown and slopping about in seven league boots, this was not much. As far as I was concerned he was enemy number one for the rest of my training.

But this wretched day was not yet over for me. A whirling, red-faced Sister flung back the doors to the theatre.

'Where's the little minx who put the leg in my bin?' I was duly pointed out. 'She's dripped all over my floor and can just come and clean it up again. Straight away.'

Too late, Alderton explained to me between giggles that an employee known as 'the meatman' came up from his department in the basement in response to a telephone call from the theatre to deal with such things as my leg.

In February 1940 our set became second year nurses with an accompanying rise in salary. We now earned £2–1–8d a month. Twelve shillings for repairs to my gramophone made a big hole in that. We were no longer the junior probationers on the wards, and I had moved up one place in the theatre. Occasionally I was allowed to take charge during a minor case in the smaller of the two theatres and I felt quite at home amongst the cupboards full of instruments whose names and functions I knew by heart. I could set out the requirements for a suprapubic cystostomy, an appendix and a ruptured ulcer. I knew each surgeon's size in gloves and the catgut he preferred.

Outside, in the real world, the fight against Hitler was becoming known as 'the phoney war'. The British Expeditionary Force in France had seen no real action yet, though Poland was lost, carved up between Germany and Russia. Sometimes we would turn our heads to see in the streets of Newcastle the unfamiliar uniform of a Polish soldier or airman who had escaped to Britain. The Free Poles, they called themselves. They must have found Newcastle strangely unconcerned about the war at that time, although enemy reconnaissance planes were seen more frequently now over the east coast and once, on my day off, I went with the crowd at Whitley Bay to view with curiosity an evil-looking spiked mine washed up there on the beach.

Then in April, with no warning, Hitler invaded Denmark and Norway. No more butter, bacon or ham would be coming to Britain from Denmark, and food rationing was intensified. Dried egg and sausages of whalemeat made their appearance. The butchers' shops were full of parsley and very little else. In the hospital, the standard of the food became even worse.

Hardly a week went by without a farewell party for a house-man or senior nurse leaving to join the Forces. Young men we had known as untidy students dazzled us in their new uniforms. Recently qualified nurses bounced back to say goodbye, swishing into the wards with that bravado that comes only when you have left the hospital for good. Anne Newsome, looking devastating in the grey and scarlet of Queen Alexandra's Imperial Military Nursing Service, made me groan with envy. It was unthinkable that the war could still be on when I would be qualified to join up, but if it was, then the army would be my choice too. Edna did not suffer from such frantic impatience. 'First things first' was her attitude and our next hurdle, the Preliminary Nursing Examination, was in twelve months' time. There was a great deal of studying to be done.

For me, it was all a means to an end but Edna would look dreamy. 'I'd really like to be a midwife,' she would say apologetically.

Scandalised, I would snap back, 'They don't want midwives in the army.'

I was moved from the theatre to the Children's Ward. This was a very different place from the children's wards of today. A great deal of well-intentioned thinking by those who laid down the rules was sadly off the mark. Visits from parents were reckoned to be upsetting for the child and so were greatly restricted. But the children could not understand why their mothers had deserted them. Nurses filled the gap so that another traumatic separation took place when the child went home. The Sister in charge was not unkind but believed it was not in the children's interest to show them affection. 'Mustn't spoil them. Makes them soft.' So, if we had a few moments to spare, we were put to sponging the leaves of the aspidistra rather than reading a fairy story.

Short stays in hospital were rare. Complete bed rest for an extended period was the norm forty years ago, during which time little white legs grew thinner and thinner and convalescence longer. Some of the children spent months in hospital. There was the eight-year-old I remember only as Charlie, who had caught his arm in a potato-peeling machine, and Mary, aged twelve, with tubercular adhesions of the intestine. Charlie, who had a spirit that could not be daunted, took a proprietary interest in the running of the ward, and while the Sister was listening to the report of the night staff, Charlie would give us his report, handing us clean pillowslips and napkins with his one good arm as we made the beds. Romances between the night nurses and medical students were his special interest and some nights he appeared to go very short of sleep. Mary was confined to bed, the disease too advanced to be checked, yet I never heard her complain. Then there were all the little girls with inflammable nighties who had burnt backs and bottoms, and had to lie on their fronts, crying with cramp and with the agony of using a bedpan. For these children, hospital meant dread of the daily dressing. I had to learn to do that, to 'scrub up' and to dress and clean a wound by the 'no touch' technique. It seemed to me at that time that there was no way of dressing burns that was not excruciatingly painful. Every dressing stuck. We tried to make up to the children afterwards, but there was always tomorrow and the dreaded sound of the dressing trolley.

I was also the 'nit nurse'. Many of the children came from poor homes where soap and water was not much in evidence, and I was soon on familiar terms with the head louse. Every morning, I went round the little beds with my bowl of disinfectant, small-toothed comb and cotton-wool swab, making sure that my own hair was well tucked away during the exercise. I saw many cases of infected glands of the neck due to an infested scalp, and when things were as bad as this, I had to shave the child's head and apply a pungent-smelling compress of oil of sassafras, which was worn like a cap for twenty-four hours. The children never seemed to mind this indignity. It was just one more inexplicable thing that happened to you in hospital.

'Great experience,' said Edna. 'Lucky you.'

The ladies on her medical ward did not have nits.

On Friday, 10th May, Hitler invaded the Netherlands. Holland fell in five days and the German army swept on, taking British and French troops completely by surprise. When the King of the Belgians capitulated, the British Expeditionary Force found itself surrounded at Dunkirk, but was able to withdraw to England, there to form a second B.E.F. Peter got his sailing orders at last, but before he could embark, France capitulated.

We expected invasion hourly. One overwrought sister thought she saw parachutes floating down over the Nurses' Home and a full-scale alarm was raised. We listened to every news bulletin on the wireless and every thundering speech by Winston Churchill. Our families at home surrendered their saucepans to make planes, and the armament factories regularly broke the records they set themselves. We pulled up garden railings to melt down for ships' plating. All the trucks and guns left behind at Dunkirk had to be replaced.

Parents made arrangements to send their children even further away to safety in Canada, but my sister, living in the beautiful valley of the North Tyne, would not let her three go. 'Better to stick together,' she said.

In July, Edna and I went back on night-duty just as the bombing raids on Britain's industrial cities began in earnest, and that included Newcastle with its shipyards. Every night, the German bombers came over. You could set your watch by the siren at eleven-thirty. The Decontamination Centre was in full use now. With the sounding of the reassuring, single note of the All Clear, ambulances came crawling up the hospital drive, bringing the injured, grey-faced from shock, with the dust of their homes in their hair, to be given transfusions and resuscitation in the Nissen hut before passing to the operating theatres and the wards.

'Give your Blood and Save a Life!' the posters urged us, and 'Dig for Victory!', 'Save for Victory!' 'Be like Dad, keep Mum!' We saved, we knitted, we made handkerchieves out of shirt tails and mittens out of old socks as Hitler plastered the country with bombs. Liverpool, Coventry, Cardiff, Bristol, Southampton and Newcastle.

We were kept busy on night-duty but at least we were able to sleep during the day. For the day-staff, every night was a broken night. Wearily, they crawled out of their beds as the siren sounded and trudged downstairs to the basement boiler room in the Nurses' Home. The boiler room was hot, the cement floor hard. Restlessly, the nurses shuffle and fidget until the first of a stick of bombs falls some distance away. The Tyne again? The next bomb is nearer and the last but one makes the pipes rattle, and rust tinkles to the ground. The nurses are back in bed by 2 a.m. and up again at 6 a.m. to wards full of last night's victims. It was South Shields last night. An air raid shelter suffered a direct hit.

My home at Whitley Bay was empty now and the windows boarded up. It was too near the mouth of the Tyne for comfort and my mother had gone to live in the country with my sister. I went to see what the bombs had done to the place where I had grown up and found that the Trinity Wesleyan Chapel had collapsed under a direct hit. The paddling pool was just a hole in the lee of a cliff and there was a gap where a school friend used to live. The only people I met on the promenade were troops watching the sea for invaders. The sands which, in other summers would have been black with day-trippers, were marked only by the trim little arrows of seagulls' feet.

In August, enemy planes which until now had attacked in tens and scores suddenly came in hundreds. Huge formations of bombers now set about destroying all our airfields, particularly those in the south and east of the country. It was the first stage of Hitler's invasion plan. After the R.A.F. was destroyed, troops would be landed from flat-bottomed barges at present under construction in the estuaries of the rivers Meuse and Scheldt. Scarcely believing what we heard, we listened to B.B.C. news commentators reporting the huge waves of enemy bombers. We went wild with excitement over numbers shot down by our fighters. We kept the score, as if it were no more lethal than a Test match, and got on with our work, re-arranging our lives where necessary to adapt to constant air raids. It was only later that we realised it had been the Battle of Britain. Terrible losses on both sides continued and it was not until the end of September that the threat of invasion finally receded. The bombing of our cities, however, went on without ceasing. We were becoming used to tragedy in the newspapers. A ship carrying children to Canada was sunk and all aboard were lost. I thought of my sister's wise decision.

Peter had been stationed in Yeovil for some time now but in October he came home with his brother Hugh on embarkation leave. They had a long trip ahead of them, round the Cape to Egypt. Mussolini had brought Italy into the war in June on Hitler's side and, with forces controlling almost the whole Mediterranean, he was now threatening Egypt.

Peter was delighted to be seeing some action at last. He had been too late for Norway and France, and he was in high spirits on the last night of his leave as we dined together at the swanky Eldon Grill in Newcastle.

The walk back to hospital was through a sadly changed city. There were many gaps now between the boarded-up shop fronts and large areas of damaged road were railed off. Giant bites had been taken out of Victorian terraces, exposing rose-papered bedrooms and absurd lavatory pedestals clinging to bare walls.

By the time we reached the hospital gates, the nightly sirens had started up and searchlights fingered the moth-like shapes of enemy planes as they emerged from behind the clouds. We said goodbye as the last notes of the siren died away, but our words were drowned in the sudden barrage from the ack-ack battery on the Moor. I hurried up the drive, turning to wave to Peter just once more. He was still standing there, a lonely figure against a crimson sky. Something was on fire down by the docks.

Inside the hospital, I joined the procession of nurses making for the basement and found that Edna had saved me a bit of bench.

'What did you have to eat?' she said.

3

The Fight for a Union

At the beginning of November, the hospital porters began agitating for a five shilling a week rise. During a debate at a branch meeting of their union, one crusading member drew attention to the poor working conditions of the nurses and enlisted a great deal of sympathy on our behalf. It was decided that one of their members would approach the hospital committee not only with their own request but also with a plea for a forty-eight hour week for the nursing staff.

The first we knew of it was a column in the *Sunday Sun* which showed the discrepancies in our working conditions compared with the other training hospital in Newcastle. We worked sixty-seven hours a week on day-duty and seventy-two on night-duty compared with the forty-eight hour week of the other hospital. For our extra hours, we were actually paid less. A first year nurse at our hospital was paid £20 a year compared with £25 at the other.

'Steps will be taken to enquire into the conditions under which the nurses work —' the union spokesman was reported to have said, and our hearts warmed to him for his interest.

For most of us, no matter what time we came off duty, whether it was a morning, afternoon or evening pass, sleep seemed the most desirable occupation and it was only with great strength of mind that we made the effort to go into the town, to see a film or visit a friend. For a great many nurses, the days went by with no break between working and sleeping.

It was very encouraging to find that a union was concerned about our welfare and it seemed to me that we should make a supporting move of some kind, so I persuaded my friends, Edna, Margaret Banks, Jean Williams, Lucy Dixon and as many others as I could impress, to write to the Editor of the *Sunday Sun*, thanking the union for its interest and corroborating the facts. I hoped that at least some would be printed.

We were rewarded by a half-page spread of letters cautiously signed – 'The Nurses', 'Three Probationers', 'The Student Nurses' etc. Excitement in the hospital was intense and action followed immediately. Three hours were knocked off our weekly total. To our great jubilation, we were now down to sixty-four hours a week. The mood was ripe for further change.

We waited, but nothing happened and slowly our confidence ebbed. We never learned the outcome of the union's appeal to the hospital committee but we did notice that we ringleaders were suddenly losing friends. The Matron, it appeared, was on the war-path, hell-bent to discover the instigators of the Press campaign, and when she found them, it was said they would be asked to leave.

Support for our reforms melted away, and now it seemed that our small group were the only nurses in the whole hospital who found anything wrong with conditions. It was suddenly bad form to mention money or the fact that we were undernourished. To do so was to tarnish the image of our selfless patron, Florence Nightingale. We withdrew, hurt, to bide our time. We could not afford to be sacked. No other hospital would accept trouble-makers.

The reforms had come to an untimely end, for there was so much still to be done. A junior nurse frequently had to wait from breakfast at 6.30 a.m. until second dinner sitting at 1.30 p.m. with only a ten minutes break at 9 a.m. in which to snatch a quick cup of tea and change into a clean apron. During this stretch from 9 a.m. to 1.30 p.m. she was not allowed to sit down for a moment nor have any further refreshment. To serve the patients' dinner when her own stomach was rumbling with emptiness was a common enough torture.

On the subject of our very poor pay, the glib response was usually that, as apprentices, we could not expect more. In this case, we argued, we should have time off for study instead of which we were required to attend all lectures in our off-duty time. This was frequently mid-morning after night-duty. Small wonder that the notes we took then were scarcely legible. Lucy Dixon fell off her chair one morning after she had had a busy night on the surgical wards. She was dead asleep. The skin specialist who was giving the lecture ticked her off roundly but did not bother to enquire why she was so tired.

All these things, and many more, irked us sorely, but the Prelim. exam was coming up fast and there were nights of intensive study ahead of us. It was no time for demonstrations yet we knew that one day we must stand up and be seen, and make our protests heard. So, to the Matron's great relief, the whole affair fizzled out and there was no more publicity about the nurses.

For once, there was better war news. We were pushing the Italians out of Libya, and in December, America passed the Lend-Lease Bill. Weapons and armaments began to flow into Britain from the United States.

1941 was the year of the Prelim. The last weeks before the dreaded date in April flew past as Edna, Margaret Banks and I bemoaned our lack of earlier application and studied long into the nights, through the sirens and the All Clears. Question and answer. Revise, revise. All the systems we had learned in the Training School were now to be taken in greater detail.

A letter came from Peter, taking two months to reach me from somewhere in the desert. Two weeks later, his sister wrote to tell me that he was dangerously ill with dysentery. She wished me luck in my examination. Nurses were not allowed to receive telephone calls, neither in the Home nor in the hospital, unless they were of an urgent nature, but on the morning of the Prelim. I was allowed to answer a call from Peggy, Peter's sister, before I went with clean cap and apron and well-sharpened pencils into the examination room. Peter was dead.

As I covered sheet after sheet of foolscap in that bare room full of chalk smells and pale Spring sunshine, I thought of the symptoms of dysentery, of Peter's lanky frame wasting away with the debilitating disease, and I could imagine his desperation as he fought a losing battle. His war had turned out to be cruelly disappointing. There is nothing heroic about dysentery.

The war dragged on. Night after night, week after week, the bombing went on. Food rations were down to the basics, but expectant mothers and babies were safeguarded against vitamin deficiency by free issues of cod liver oil, rose-hip syrup and concentrated orange juice. All our clothing was rationed. We needed coupons for handkerchieves, stockings, sheets, furniture and sweets. There was a brisk trade in old parachutes which we made into underwear of a sort; very slippery, unsympathetic pants they made, and of a hideous sharp yellow, but at least they required no coupons. A letter for me one morning addressed in Peter's big, bold handwriting made my heart turn over. It had been written three weeks before he died.

With the Prelim. successfully behind us, Edna and I were once more on night-duty. To my delight, I was sent back to the theatre, my old stamping ground, but this time I was in charge and had a junior nurse to help me. It was a calm place by night, free from histrionics, and the registrars and housemen who operated were old friends. Russell Slater and Ray Dobson, newly qualified and awaiting call-up, did some of the minor surgery and sat with us throughout many an air raid as the junior nurse and I patched gloves in the anteroom by the dim light of a hurricane lamp. As soon as the All Clear sounded, we sprang into action; lights up, instruments ready, for operating would begin shortly after the arrival of the first casualties. It was unsafe for ambulances to make the journey to the hospital during an alert and civilian emergencies were often unfortunately delayed because of this. We waited for most of one night for a poor soul with a ruptured ulcer who had been caught in a succession of raids. Nights like these were hard on the surgeons who could not easily replace their lost sleep.

One of the registrars, genial, shaggy Mr. Stanley Raw came back one day as Capt. Raw, R.A.M.C., to bid us goodbye, and we hardly recognized him. Bulging pockets and baggy trousers had been replaced by well-cut khaki and shiny Sam Browne.

'How handsome he is,' we sighed.

'Nonsense,' said the student dressers. 'It's only the uniform.'

When it was his turn to go, even Russell Slater contrived to look elegant in the uniform of a surgeon-lieutenant of the Royal

Naval Reserve. 'Family tradition,' he explained. 'Great grand-father was a butcher aboard an East-Indiaman.'

By the time we were back on day-duty, Edna and I were beginning to reconsider those long postponed reforms. Nothing further had been done since the Matron's first panicky gesture of knocking three hours from our working week. We decided to approach the union which had originally interested itself on our behalf, the National Union of General and Municipal Workers, and to ask for their advice. They sent us Mr. Esther.

We met him, Edna, Margaret Banks, Lucy Dixon and I, in the Haymarket Cafe one evening, and found that he was not our cup of tea at all, too full of doctrines about 'the workers' and our fight against 'Them'. This was not how we saw the problem. We were asking for better conditions for nurses, and were not interested in ideas about society in general, but it seemed that Mr. Esther and his union were the only allies we had.

He generously bought each of us a plate of fish and chips. We would have liked to decline, but our empty stomachs shouted louder than our principles and we scoffed it all, watched bene-volently by Mr. Esther, who was not hungry.

The problem, it was explained to us, was that the nurses made little effort to help themselves. No outside help could be given if the nurses did not seek it.

He had with him, as it happened, details of a registered Nurses' Guild which had considerable bargaining weight. Now, if we could persuade one third of the total number of nurses at the hospital to become members of the Guild, then representation on our behalf could be made to the house committee. Selected nurses would then, by right, sit in at the meetings and we would have a platform for airing our griev-ances. Edna saw the practical difficulties.

'What happens if Matron gives us the sack for causing trouble? She was wild enough about the letters.'

Mr. Esther packed his pipe importantly.

'If you adopt the right procedure, you'll be protected by the union.'

We thanked him and went thoughtfully back to the hospital.

The first step ahead of us was the worst step. Matron must be told of our intention to form a union and she would not like that at all.

'Her answer will be that we already have the Royal College of Nursing to legislate for us.' Margaret was beginning to have doubts.

'The R.C.N. is a dead duck,' I said. This was true in those days, in 1941, before the light of change illuminated that austere body, before enquiries were made into the nursing service and before the Whitley Report. 'What has it ever done for us?' I demanded.

Once we had decided to go ahead, we four began to spread the word about, and this time, perhaps because we were all senior nurses now, we drummed up considerable interest. It seemed that there would be good support for our crusade so we wrote to Mr. Esther telling him we were about to launch the Guild and to take the first step, that is, inform the Matron.

I had known from the very beginning that the agony of facing the Matron would be mine. The whole movement had been my idea so there was no passing the buck for this next, particularly unattractive undertaking.

I put on a clean cap and apron and mounted the stairs to the Matron's office to take my place at the end of a line of nurses apprehensively waiting to pay a fine of 2/6d. for breaking a thermometer (approximately six per cent of their monthly salary). My mouth was dry and my heart thumped. I had never felt so frightened before, and my inside turned over when, in answer to my knock, the omnipotent, plump little figure, all starch and cleanliness, called out in her high-pitched voice to come in.

I did not like the way she looked at me, her mouth pursed, her eyes raking my uniform for faults. It was clear I had no ally here. What exactly did I do if she gave me the sack? There would be no references, that was certain. Mr. Esther had said: 'The union will stand behind you.' Well, they were not behind me right now and she was waiting for me to begin.

In as firm a voice as I could muster, I announced that it was the intention of a group of nurses to start a branch of The Nurses' Guild at the hospital. I stopped and waited. It took a minute for the outrageous statement to sink in.

The Matron's eyes widened in disbelief. Her knuckles resting on the desk whitened and her pencil snapped in half.

I stood firm, drawing strength from the fact that I was now up to my neck in it anyway and had nothing more to lose. I tried to keep my voice steady as I suggested that we nurses felt some improvement in our conditions was overdue. She became very angry indeed and the starched white bow under her dimpled chin wobbled in her agitation.

'I'll soon put a stop to that!' she shouted, and there was a sudden silence amongst the shuffling crowd outside. 'Get out!' She flung out her little pink hand towards the door. 'Get back to your work!' and she banged on the desk, making all the papers bounce, frightening her fat cat out of its wits. The cat and I retreated together, with me trying to retain some dignity, but my hand was trembling as I closed the door behind me. The silent line of nurses waiting outside looked at me, aghast and shaken.

'I've got to go to the lav,' murmured the next in line and fled down the corridor.

With their eyes upon me, I made what I hoped was a stately descent down the stone stairs and returned to the ward, my mind in a turmoil. An irrevocable step had been taken. There was to be a meeting of the Big Four in my room that night, after duty.

Predictably, open war was now declared between those in authority and us, the acknowledged ringleaders. Our faith in Mr. Esther was not misplaced however. He was right when he said there were no legitimate grounds for dismissal in our actions so far. The Matron must have discovered this, for we were marked down for close observation on our wards. The Ward Sisters watched us like hawks for any faults which could serve as an excuse for dismissal and we had to be extra careful.

But the Guild was launched. Members were needed now as quickly as possible so that we could be recognized by the Union of General and Municipal Workers and given legal teeth. We spread the word every night after duty. Without a scruple, I harangued the latest intake from the Training School. They were so raw they did not know what they were signing, but signatures and the sixpence-a-month union fees were essential. We drew a lot of support from the nurses of our year and the year junior to us but the more senior nurses were too near their Finals to worry much about conditions. There were three hundred nurses on the staff so we had to get one hundred signatures.

'You'll never get a hundred signatures!' the Matron screamed at me, but we did.

Our self-appointed committee consisted of Edna as Treasurer; myself as Secretary; Lucy as Recruitment Officer, and Margaret and a fiery red-head named Gilroy in a vague office known as 'liaison'. We drew up the list of members, entered up our funds and sent a formal notification via Mr. Esther to the Nurses' Guild. We were off.

From then on, it was easier going because we now had the backing of an outside body which the hospital had to acknowledge, albeit reluctantly. These were the days before the National Health Service. The Royal Victoria Infirmary was a voluntary hospital, that is, it was supported by contributions from the local community, particularly from the miners who did not begrudge the few pence taken from their weekly pay packet. Each one knew that the chance of finding himself a patient at the hospital were very high at any time. Because of their considerable financial support, elected working men, miners mostly, attended the regular House Committee meetings held in the hospital and chaired by Sir Ralph Mortimer. There was no spokesman for the nurses. Now, at the request of our union, a representative nurse for each of the four years' of training was invited to attend. Gilroy represented fourth year, myself, third year, and we found two articulate junior reformers in first and second years.

When we took our seats for the first time there were no welcoming speeches from the top table where Matron sat with

Sir Ralph and his secretary, but we soon found that the little body of miners sitting opposite us in their best navy-blue suits, were the staunchest allies we could wish for. They would not allow us to be steam-rollered by the rhetoric of the governing body. We began to whittle away at our grievances.

I was particularly concerned about lack of rations on a nurse's day off. Whenever we went home, it was with empty hands. We were eating someone else's share of the tiny weekly allowance of butter, sugar, meat, tea and cheese. Members of the Forces were issued with temporary ration coupons when on leave, even if it was only for a day, which were included in the allocations of the household thus making a small but significant contribution. I could not see why the same arrangement should not apply to us. As it was, the hospital benefitted every time a nurse was absent from a meal.

Sir Ralph and I had a head-on collision on this point.

'Do you suppose my friends expect me to bring a ration book when they invite me to dinner?' he asked weightily, accompanied by supportive murmurs from the Matron and the secretary.

I had done my homework properly. 'A nurse's day off covers: one dinner, two suppers, one breakfast and one tea. To accept all that and make no contribution would be surely as distasteful to you as it is to us ... sir.' We got our ration coupons and earned the gratitude of three hundred nurses' Mums.

We brought other points to the notice of the House Committee. An inspection of the hospital kitchens was made after our cold brisket was found to be crawling with maggots. Another of our grievances was that although an allowance for board and lodging was deducted from our salary, it was not replaced in holiday pay. Mr. Esther put us up to this one.

For years we had been too trusting to question such things, but now we had a voice and we proceeded to make ourselves heard. We achieved an allowance of ten shillings and sixpence per week for board and lodgings while on holiday, which, though not a fat sum, was better than nothing.

On a 6–10 p.m. pass, if a nurse did not choose to return for the regular hospital supper at 9 p.m., there was nothing for her to eat until breakfast next morning, not even the possibility of a sandwich or a hot drink unless she could beg, borrow or steal a spoonful of tea to brew her own. From now on, a large pot of coffee was left on the hotplate in the dining-room along with any left-overs from supper, for the benefit of nurses on an evening pass. All these concessions seem small now, so many years later, but at the time, we greeted them like the dawn of a new liberality.

As a union, the Nurses' Guild was a poor, weak thing but it served to set the ball rolling and eventually forced the legitimate Royal College of Nursing to examine more closely the conditions under which nurses worked. The Guild faded away and today our struggle at the Royal Victoria Infirmary is quite forgotten. Nurses there are obviously happy at their work and relations with the administrative staff are relaxed and friendly. No-one is hungry any more. The dining-room with its hallowed procedures has given way to a self-service cafeteria. No night nurses struggle to concentrate over mid-morning lectures now. There are recognised study periods through a syllabus in which standards are being constantly raised.

Forty years ago, we could not see the light ahead, but the slight rewards we achieved seemed a sweet breath of promise to all of us who were trying to hang on to the end of four punishing years.

Three years to the day, we reported to the Linen Room to be measured for 'Greys', as the blue frocks of Staff Nurses were inexplicably called, and my next position was as junior Staff Nurse, back on the Children's Ward, back to those burns, to nappies, wet beds, prayers at night and Syrup of Figs. This time, I was no longer the 'nit nurse'.

It was 1942 and the army nursing service was only one year ahead of me now while the war was no nearer a conclusion. In fact, the scene was more confused than ever. The bombing of Pearl Harbour had brought the Americans into the conflict, and Germany's attack on Russia had given Britain a strange ally.

Throughout that year, we prepared for our Final examination, and all our experiences on the wards and long hours of study were put to the test in April 1943. Margaret, Edna and I celebrated our success with a 4/6d. bottle of Sandeman's sherry after duty in my room. We made such a noise that we brought the Home Sister to the door, saying didn't we know it was after 'Lights Out' and who was that under the bed? But Edna could not come out because she had caught her curlers in the wire mattress and, in any case, nothing mattered any more. We were State Registered Nurses. Edna and Margaret decided to do Part One midwifery before following me into the army. Lucy Dixon and Jean Williams chose the Navy – and we split up.

The free world was clamouring for a Second Front, a landing to be launched by the Allies somewhere in Europe, to drive Hitler from the occupied countries. All over Britain, the words 'SECOND FRONT NOW!' were chalked on hoardings, walls and bridges.

At my interview in the War Office building in Newcastle, a matron of the Queen Alexandra's Imperial Military Nursing Service/Reserve, who carried a crown on her shoulder, regarded me soberly with a steady, non-committal gaze. Was I prepared to travel overseas in conditions which might be far from comfortable?

'Yes, Ma'am,' I told her. I would travel anywhere.

On 27th September, 1943, I was posted to the 75th British General Hospital in Peebles, Scotland, as Nursing Officer B. McBryde. Q.A.I.M.N.S/R. Personal number P/294203.

Part II

4

Q.A.I.M.N.S/R.

I arrived at Peebles on a sunny, autumn afternoon when maple and mountain ash flamed on the surrounding hills. At first sight, from the window of the taxi that was bringing me from the station, I fell in love with the sturdy little town.

There were signs of welcome everywhere; whist drives and a Saturday Night Hop at the Assembly Hall, coffee and buns at The Forces' Canteen, home-made scones and a pot of tea at The Tea Room run by the Women's Voluntary Service. Gentians were on the tables, as blue as the September sky, and a soft-spoken lady in hand-knits waited to welcome every member of H.M. Forces.

With three other new arrivals, I was on my way to the Hydro, which in peacetime was a respectable and rather grand hotel but was now a military hospital. We were four nurses knowing nothing about each other except what we had picked up during the train journey north. Mary Smith was from Rugby. Her reserve was yet to thaw out. Helen Souter was a Mancunian Scot, bubbling with good spirits, dimpled and chubby; and Margaret Kilduff, a dreamy-eyed, graceful girl, came from Leicester. I, whose head went straight into my shoulders, envied her long neck.

The taxi put us down outside a handsome, gabled building with balustrades, commanding magnificent views on all sides. Servicemen in shirt sleeves were hosing down drab military ambulances where, no doubt, uniformed chauffeurs had dusted their Rolls in peacetime. A sergeant who was supervising the erection of tents on the tennis courts turned to stare at us, four civilians, cluttered with handbags, holdalls and raincoats, reporting for a first army posting. We climbed the steps to the main entrance and went inside.

There was very little left to remind one of the peace-time

hotel. Army boots clattered over empty floors. The ballroom bristled with the Tobruk plasters and the Balkan Beams
of an orthopaedic ward. The honeymoon suite was an
operating theatre. Daily Orders hung in the place of the Menu
of the Day and a nuggetty clerk in khaki manned the reception
desk.

'If you'll come with me, Sisters, I'll show you your quarters.'
We were all sisters now. The transformation from civilian
nursing had begun.

Our first few days were taken up with inoculations and medi-
cal examinations. The first army nursing sister I met was Sarah
Parsons. Tall, blonde and very beautiful in a crisp white head
veil, she stood reassuringly by my side while Capt. Lloyd,
R.A.M.C. tapped my reflexes and peered down my throat.
Sarah was one of our few married sisters. Her husband was an
M.O. with the Long Range Desert Group in Africa.

A trip to Edinburgh to buy kit followed and the shopping list
was formidable; an ant-proof tin trunk that in itself carried
sinister implications; a folding camp-bed and a bedroll or
'valise'; a canvas wash bowl on a tripod; a collapsible canvas
bath; a canvas bucket; a 'Beatrice' paraffin stove and a pair of
gumboots. It was all good, pioneering stuff.

Next, the uniform. A well-cut grey suit and greatcoat, both
with scarlet facings, tailored for us by Austin Reed, pearl-grey
shirts and matching ties. On duty we wore a grey cotton frock
with shoulder cape trimmed with scarlet, and on our heads, a
veil of fine lawn. It would take all next month's salary to pay the
bill for this shopping spree but army pay was munificent after
the miserable pittance of our training days. For the first time in
my life I needed a cheque book.

Once out of our civilian clothes, we were swallowed without
trace in the Sisters' Mess of the 75th British General Hospital
(B.G.H.). For most of us, it was a first army appointment but
some had seen several years' service in the Middle East and the
two 'regulars', with service in peace and war, were superior
beings indeed. One of these sisters, Miss Agate, had three pips
up, and the reputation of being able to organise an efficient

theatre in a hen-run if necessary. The 'Miss' was never dropped out of respect for that extra pip.

The life was very different from nursing in a civilian hospital. Work on the wards involved a great deal of form-filling. There was an army regulation, it seemed, for every situation, and for every situation there was a corresponding form to be filled in. The old hands rattled them off in a most confusing way. 'You'll want a B 29 for that and an A 56 for the other.' The surgeon who asked me for a D 66 would have got what he wanted much more quickly if he'd asked for an X-Ray form, but one became accustomed to the system and it worked.

The absence of any female patients seemed strange at first. There were no nighties or talcum powder, no arguments over who owned which flowers. These were no-nonsense wards, with striped pyjamas and parade-ground lockers. There was a photograph of the regulation lay-out for a locker with towel folded in three and shaving gear just so, and this is how it had to be for the daily round of the commanding officer, Colonel H. J. G. Wells. All the orderlies were male and clumped about in big boots, wearing a white smock over their khaki, while we Q.A.s, butterflying about in our starched white veils, were the only women in this very male assembly.

Work was unhurried, with plenty of staff to deal with the bronchitis and pneumonia of the medical wards, traffic accidents and hernias of the surgical department. There was a sprinkling of long-term cases dating back to Dunkirk. I wrote to Edna who was cycling in the wake of a trained midwife around 'the district'. She had just delivered her first baby.

'Better you than me,' I wrote. 'It would put me off for ever. The army's great,' I added.

Our hospital unit, raw and ragged after a large recent intake of personnel, was in the process of sorting itself out. Doctors, sisters and orderlies were learning to work together. Right from the first day, we became aware of an undercurrent of excitement running through the hospital. Rumours about the Second Front were rife. It was commonly believed that our unit was to take part in the campaign, wherever that might be, and the guesses were legion. Norway? Denmark? Calais? Marseilles? Italy perhaps?

Colonel Wells walked ponderously about the tidy wards, inspecting lockers, kitchen sinks, urinals and pig swill. 'Things are moving fast,' he would say mysteriously. 'Things are on the move.' Then he would pass on, leaving a question in the air.

'He's been saying that ever since I came to Scotland six months ago.' Miss Agate squashed all conjecture. 'So don't get carried away.'

In our third week at the Hydro, the entire company of sisters was handed over to Regimental Sergeant Major Regan to be toughened up. It was quite obvious that he regarded us as a useless, over-indulged bunch of women.

'Right then,' he announced. 'Route march. Gas masks. Tin hats. Nursing Officers for the training of. See what you're made of.'

He led us, wearing khaki slacks, battledress jackets and tin hats, with gas haversacks on our backs, up the side of the fell and down again. It was only five miles but it felt like twenty. With slacks covered in mud and bits of bracken, we arrived back at the Hydro to face his scorn. We were struggling for breath while he, maddeningly, showed no sign of fatigue or exertion. The crease in his trousers was still knife-edged and the toes of his big, black boots shone like a pair of bowler's woods.

A grin split his face. 'My, my. We are in a state. We shall have to take ourselves in hand, shan't we? A few exercises to get rid of that flabby fat. Can't have our Nursing Officers letting the side down when the 75th goes over the top.'

A cold, precise Edinburgh accent near me. Margaret Anderson had just got her breath back. 'I hope, Sergeant Major,' she said, 'should you be so unfortunate as to fall ill, that it may be my privilege to nurse you.'

Discomfiture darkened his leathery face and to roars of applause he turned on his cracker-jack heel and headed for the Sergeants' Mess.

Self-defence was the next useful skill we had to learn; how to tip up an assailant from behind and what could be done with the sharp edge of a heel. The hospital buzzed with instruction. When we were not actually nursing, we were learning how to keep medical records in the field, how to purify water, the lay-out of a general hospital under canvas, how the field kitchen worked, the functions of the padre on active service.

We became familiar with the progress of a wounded man from the time he was picked up by stretcher-bearers and hurried to his Regimental Aid Post (R.A.P.) then taken by ambulance to the Field Dressing Station (F.D.S.) or Casualty Clearing Station (C.C.S.) for urgent surgery, then down the line to the base hospitals of which the 75th British General was one. Here he would receive treatment before being evacuated by sea or air to the United Kingdom or sent back for service with his company. In our 600 bedded hospital unit there was a mobile X-Ray section, pathology and dental departments, surgical and medical wards, a resuscitation centre, an operating theatre and ancillary offices. We were a self-contained medical unit.

We attended lectures on typical battle injuries and how they should be treated. Lt. Colonel Harding, i/c Surgical Division, flashed a confident eye over his hushed audience. 'If the man has been shot through the popliteal vein and his foot is cold and gangrenous, don't waste time. Cut it off.' There was a profound silence. I nervously reflected upon the state of my scissors. There was no dropping off to sleep during *these* lectures.

Captain Johnson, the dental officer, a quiet, gentle man, spoke next. 'Fractured jaw,' he began. 'Treat for shock. Pick out any loose teeth and bits of bone then put a stitch through the tongue and tie it to a button on his jacket before you send him down the line on a stretcher.' His audience winced. Civvy nursing was never like this. These notes were probably intended for medical officers originally but they startled us into thinking objectively about the kind of nursing we might expect on active service.

Autumn gave way to a more wintry landscape and snow capped the hills behind the Hydro. We bought woollen spencers to wear under our cotton uniforms and gave out extra blankets in the wards. Mary Smith, the girl from Rugby who had now come by the nickname of 'Pin', approached me one day. A six weeks' course in plastic surgery was being offered to two sisters. Should she put our names down? Work on the overstaffed wards was not particularly demanding just then, so we went ahead and applied for the course which was to be held at a nearby Burns Unit.

The burns centre at Bangour had come into being as a result of the Battle of Britain in 1940 when so many airmen had been badly burned. After their initial treatment had come the need for plastic surgery, to free joints from binding scar tissue, to build up new faces again. Here, in Bangour, the work of repair was still going on for some of those Battle of Britain pilots. The unit, built as an emergency hospital, sprawled up a bleak hillside in single-storey, wooden buildings. Pin and I were given a room each in a hut allotted to the civilian staff and were made welcome by the Scottish girls there. That first morning, when we accompanied the surgeons (Mr. Wallis and Mr. Buchan) and their physiotherapists around the wards, was a revelation to us both.

The scarred hands of one R.A.F. pilot were contracted back towards the wrist to a position where they were virtually functionless. His face was young and handsome but his raw, red hands were like bunches of boiled prawns.

Mr. Wallis pointed to the tough cords at the wrist that were immobilising the hands. 'We'll remove all this scar tissue, straighten out the wrist, skin graft the raw area and wrap the whole thing in plaster till it heals. OK?'

The owner of the hands nodded enthusiastically. As I sketched a diagram in my notebook, it dawned on me that this man was injured in 1940. It was now 1943 and hospital treatment still stretched for months, maybe years, ahead for him.

The next patient was sitting with a bundle of cane on his lap and the beginnings of a basket. He was one of the success stories, we were told, but to Pin and me he looked like a major disaster. Three years ago, he had leapt from his burning, spiralling plane, a little knot of flame at the end of a parachute. His limbs were mobile now but his face was still in the process of being rebuilt. The new eyelids were still puffy, still showing the stitchmarks, and the large, round graft on one cheek was the pale skin from his left buttock that had not yet taken on colour from the face's blood supply. Twin tunnels in a stub of bone was all he had left of a nose. Mindful that our reactions, as new-comers, were being closely observed by these patients, Pin and I were careful to show no emotion.

The surgeon was describing to us the repair he had carried out on the pilot's mouth. 'Contracting muscle was pulling it right over here to the other side of his face and we're very pleased with the correction.'

'That goes for me, too,' said Pilot Officer Humphrey, who still needed lips.

'What we did,' the surgeon went on, 'was to strip a length of fascia from his leg muscle and insert one end here, stitching it to the corner of his mouth. Then we made another incision here by the cheekbone on the same side of the face, inserted long sinus forceps to the corner of the mouth to pick up the free end of the fascia strip, pulled it through and secured it. Now he can smile.'

I tried to nod intelligently and wondered with despair what Mr. Humphrey could find to smile about. He was listening intently to everything the surgeon was saying.

'And now we'll tackle your nose.' The junior surgeon Mr. Buchan took the top off his pen and made a note in his pocket book.

'Great!' said the airman. 'Give me something to blow for Christmas.'

The surgeons bent over Mr. Humphrey with a skin-marking pencil and sketched a diagram on his forehead. 'There's good skin here and a good hair line. We'll swing down a flap incor-porating some hair-bearing cells which will be used for nostrils later. The raw area on the forehead will be grafted from the abdomen.'

So it went on, all around the ward, robbing Peter to pay Paul, taking skin from undamaged areas to graft on to denuded places, sometimes planting little islets of skin, leaving them to grow and unite. This was surgery calling for great patience on the part of surgeon and patient alike, with many trips to the operating theatre before the job was finished.

Then we came to the pedicle grafts, known amongst the men themselves as the 'dangle'ums', which was self-explanatory at a certain stage of the repair. Aircraftsman Harding was in the process of receiving a pedicle graft to the badly scarred right side of his face. A tube of flesh had been formed on the calf of one leg by stitching together two sides of an incised rectangle. When the blood supply was established within this tube, one end was freed from the leg and stitched to the palm of the hand. Again, time was allowed for a blood supply to be established between the palm of the hand and the end of the flesh tube, then that end which was still attached to the calf was freed, trimmed to fit and stitched over the burnt area of the face. The patient now had a bridge of flesh between his cheek and his palm and this remained until the cheek itself was seen to be involved in the circulation. Then the tube of flesh was removed from the hand and the hand grafted. Now the patient had earned the title of 'Dangle'um' for a pedicle of flesh hung from cheek, or nose or whatever was being repaired. They made a weird but valiant group, forming themselves into the Dangle'Ums' Club with a special membership badge. When the pedicle was seen to have a healthy blood supply from the face, it was trimmed and moulded to make a flesh cheek or nose, a result which could not have been achieved with a thin graft.

Up to now, I'd thought of plastic surgery in connection with face-lifts for aging women. Bangour showed me its real purpose. There were men with burnt elbows stitched inside the raised skin of the abdomen, immobilised there until the graft should 'take'. New lower jaws were fashioned from bottom ribs. Uppers of burnt feet were stitched to the underside of calves. Men with extensive body burns were lowered into warm saline baths and encouraged by physiotherapists to keep muscles flexible with the gentle movements possible under the water. Dressings here did not stick. I remembered my burnt children at Newcastle.

Pin and I, in theatre clothing, stood by the operating table while the surgeons sewed gossamer stitches on skin no stronger than the skim on boiled milk, heads bent, working slowly and patiently, sometimes for two hours at a stretch. They encouraged our interest, demonstrating the dermatome, a roller-type instrument for removing skin, and they showed us how the grafts must be dressed. After the initial treatment in the theatre when the grafts were firmly fixed in position by bandages or by plaster of Paris, it was six to ten days before the first dressing was done, depending on the thickness of the skin used. This was a job for either Pin or myself and was always a tense moment. If the graft had 'taken', the patient could move on to the next stage; if not, the operation would have to be repeated at a future date and that would mean more raw donor areas, leaving less skin for grafting.

To remove the last covering and see a dry, healthy graft was as exciting for us as for the patient. If part of the graft had sloughed off and there was pus, then four-hourly saline packs had to be applied and a swab sent to the pathology department. This was a technique new to us. An infected wound was always investigated for the culprit organism and then treated specifically; elementary, one might think, but not standard practice. We filled a notebook with the classification of harmful bacteria and their neutralisers. We learned to remove stitches with delicacy where a shaky hand could undo the miracle worked by the surgeon. We learned the absolute necessity of irrigation after food on stitchlines in the mouth. Minced chicken adhering to a repair of soft palate was no good to anyone. There was a whole new range of instruments for us to memorise, named after their innovators; McIndoe's fine, tapering dissecting forceps, Gillies' rake retractor, Gillies' needleholder with cutting edge, and many more. This was a new and fascinating field of surgery and the day we removed the plaster from those previously contracted wrists of the pilot was one of the many sublime moments of success. We had seen the operation to free his hands of restricting bands of scar tissue. We had watched while a dermatome graft was applied to the now extended wrists. Now, one week later, it was time to see the result.

There was a bad smell as we cut through the plaster. The airman's nostrils quivered. We removed the cotton wool, the acriflavine gauze and the tulle gras underneath. Slowly, we uncovered a pink, dry graft with only a very small area of subcutaneous haemorrhage. The graft was totally successful and the new, extended position of the wrists a great improvement. His hands could now be made to work. There was some swelling due to the plaster but the physiotherapist was already dealing with that. It was a moment of acute satisfaction for everyone concerned.

Time passed quickly. Christmas came and was made much of, with free beer, a film show, turkey and pudding. My 'plastic' Christmas was one of the happiest I have ever spent in hospital. Pin was a wonderful nurse. All her natural shyness left her when she was caring for these men. I would look across the ward and see her face lit up as she jollied along some brave buffoon in a paper cap above his own false nose. We kept our pity for when we were alone.

If one were to judge from the general hilarity of the men, it would seem that no-one there had a care in the world. One or two went home to their families for the holiday but the majority of these dreadfully mutilated men preferred to stay in hospital and I wondered if the wards, with their freakish inhabitants, had indeed become the real world. New noses, ears and chins were something to boast about here but the outside world could be cruelly inquisitive or too politely ignoring. Out there, they would have to accept sly glances from fellow travellers on the buses, peeps from behind the neighbours' curtains and piercing announcements from small children.

We were back at the Hydro in time for Hogmanay with heads and notebooks full of this new kind of nursing. Helen Souter was emerging as a first class forager. With New Year's Eve almost upon us, she had established useful contacts with the teetotallers of the unit and had acquired several surplus N.A.A.F.I. rations of booze and cigarettes.

'She amazes me,' Margaret Kilduff recounted Soutie's activities. 'Should have been a quartermaster.'

There were all the ingredients for a proper celebration of the new year. The Sergeants' Mess laid on a barrel of beer, and a piper from the town was to lead a first-footing party. Our sick Polish officers were confused. 'What about the other foot?'

There were Polish units near the hospital made up of men who had escaped when Hitler and Russia overran their country. As an ethnic experiment, it was a great success. They settled in happily alongside the Scots. We had several as patients at the time and found them very entertaining. They were unquestionably brave and quite fearless yet surprised us by wearing hair nets at night as they slept.

1944 came in with enthusiasm and optimism. Everyone knew that this would be the year of the Second Front.

5

The Second Front

Entire company to report this day 1800 hrs.
Concert hall.
Signed
H. J. G. Wells. Commanding Officer.

The chit of paper flapped in the draught. A steadying hand
went up from the crowd around the notice board and the word
passed around that this was something big. The Old Man did
not address the unit *en masse* unless he had something important
to communicate. We waited for the appointed hour with
impatience. With five minutes to go, the old concert hall, once
the setting for string ensembles amongst the potted palms, was
packed to the doors. The complete unit was there, doctors,
sisters, orderlies, clerks, cooks and drivers. On the dot of six
o'clock, the C.O. came into the hall. The buzz of conversation
died away and he mounted the stairs to the platform in perfect
silence, standing there, quite still, while the doors to the hall
were locked and a guard posted outside.

He cleared his throat. 'I am able to tell you now,' he said, a
bit choky, not at all his usual self, 'that this hospital is to play a
notable part in the next campaign of the war.' Excitement
gripped each one of us. We were to be in the Second Front. I
felt a warm, prideful feeling to be part of this unit. We were one
piece of a larger pattern that would soon be taking shape.

The C.O. was speaking again. 'At the moment, all you need
to know is that we hand over this hospital in two days' time to
the 106 General. We move to another location to pack and crate
our equipment ready for shipping.'

His eye wandered speculatively over us. He must have been
wondering what kind of a bunch we were. He barely knew some
of the recent arrivals and he was probably wondering how we

would stand up to whatever lay ahead. So was I. I even felt a twinge of gratitude towards the R.S.M. for his efforts to toughen us up.

'We entrain 0800 hrs, 10th January. I do not need to remind you that this information is top secret.'

And that was all. The Old Man stepped down from the platform and the doors were unlocked. Thoughtfully, we broke up and wandered off. The chance was coming to finish the war off at last, after four and a half long years, the war Peter had said would be over in three months, that had claimed his life and that of so many others.

Margaret Kilduff and I went for a last walk over the fells.

'We'll miss dear old Peebles,' said Duff as we climbed the rough path together. She had a way of walking with her head always a little in front, nose up, as if there was something delicious waiting for us at the crest of the hill.

'The smoky old Snug at the Cleikum,' I sighed.

'Beetle Drives at the Assembly Hall.'

There had been several light falls of snow over the last few days and we could see sheep scratching about for vegetation on the other side of the straggling, dry-stone walls, making dark holes in the white blanket. Suddenly we stopped, our attention rivetted on a metal object sticking out from the snow not far from the sheep. We regarded it in silence for a few moments. Finally Duff said with conviction, 'It's a butterfly bomb.'

On a Ministry of Information film shown to the unit the previous night, we had seen this new anti-personnel bomb that Hitler was scattering at random over Britain. Several had already been recovered from nearby hills and we had been warned to keep a sharp look-out for them. The nose of this one lay buried in the snow while the tail, consisting of two parallel rods of metal joined at the end, projected some ten inches from the ground. It was obvious to both of us that the sheep must be protected. There were a lot of meat rations walking around there. We took stones from part of the wall by the lane and built a barricade around the bomb, then hurried back to Peebles, to report our discovery.

Not only did we impress the local policeman but half the town got to hear of the bomb and a black line of people followed at a discreet distance as we led the way back up the hill.

'Wha's all this, then?' asked the policeman sternly as we approached the gap we had made in the wall. 'Who's bashed the wall doon?'

We hastened to reassure him and pointed with quiet pride to the walled-off bomb. 'We made sure the sheep didn't get hurt.' Certainly there were no sheep near the bomb. In fact there were no sheep anywhere. They seemed to have gone elsewhere.

The people from the town had quietly moved up around us, expectation written on their faces as our brave policeman strode through the gap in the wall and looked over the barricade. There was a gasp of alarm as he carelessly threw one leg over, bringing down a hail of stones, but more bravado was to follow. We watched in disbelief as the foolhardy young man grabbed the bomb by the tail and wrenched it out of the earth.

'Is this your bomb?' he said tersely, looking straight at Duff and me. There was a murmur behind us. The phlegmatic Scottish faces permitted themselves a smile and we were suddenly assailed by doubt.

'It's naught but a mole-trap, dearie. These ways are full of them.'

Our policeman caught a handful of boys before they could join the rest of the dispersing crowd. 'You laddies run up the lane and find them sheep. If Andrew Ropson finds his wall doon and all his sheep gone, he'll skelp the lot of us.'

Early on the morning of the 10th January, the unit formed up outside the Hydro to march to the station. We had said goodbye to our patients and handed them over to the relieving hospital. Trucks carrying our gear went ahead, cautiously negotiating the icy surface of the road, and now we picked up our feet to the command of the Company Officer, Lieut. Smith, setting off in as military fashion as we could manage so that we should not let the unit down. Our general bearing had certainly improved since those first days but there was still too much bobbing up and down and too much hip-swinging for R.S.M. Regan's critical eye.

A surprise awaited the company. As we swung out of the main gates of the Hydro, we were greeted by the Peebles Pipe Band which had turned out specially on this top-secret occasion to escort us to the station and give us a royal farewell, with all the townsfolk out on the streets to wave us on. Even our policeman had a smile for us and a smart salute as we passed his station.

Right to the platform, the pipes kept up their stirring march then slid into a mournful 'Will ye no' come back again?' as the train left the station with arms waving from every window.

St. Agatha's Orphanage in Watford was a Victorian-Gothic monster, a place of sooty pinnacles and thick, brown paint, drainpipes and dusty laurels. The children who normally lived there had been evacuated and, for them, the change could only have been beneficial.

Here we were to pack field equipment, and the job was waiting for us when we arrived from Peebles. Bales of straw, sacking, cans of paint, wooden crates and tins of smelly brown grease were all stacked in the Great Hall. Each piece of hospital equipment was to be wrapped, labelled and crated in category so that the whole could be reassembled with the minimum of delay 'over there', wherever that might be. Each surgical instrument had to be greased to prevent rust, wrapped in oiled paper, sewn in sacking and packed in crates which were then stencilled with an identifying number. Our fingers grew sore from sewing the coarse sacking and the stink of lubricating grease pervaded our hair, skin and clothes. After a few days, the Great Hall began to look like some mediaeval workshop with figures hammering, painting, sewing. Over our heads, clouds of dust and fluff from the sacking gyrated lazily in the pale February sunlight as we packed our hospital in preparation for the Second Front.

At last the job was finished and there was a breathing space for us to repair broken nails and remove paint marks from clothing. There was a chance for us to visit London, only thirty-five minutes away in the Tube. It was a sobering experience. There were holes as big as quarries where buildings had once

stood and demolition squads were at work, bringing down tot-
tering walls in clouds of dust. Yet there was a vitality in the
streets that one could not help noticing. We rubbed shoulders
with a score of different uniforms, square-hatted Czechs,
Poles, Norwegian sailors, Free French and all the Common-
wealth representatives. The pavement outside the Rainbow
Room in Piccadilly was six deep in American G.I.s. They stared
curiously at us, not familiar with our grey and scarlet.

'Are you Russian or Salvation Army?' they asked an indig-
nant Pin.

Slogans were painted everywhere. 'Second Front Now!' All
of us in uniform who crowded around Swan and Edgar's and
fed the pigeons in Trafalgar Square shared the secret knowledge
that the time was not very far away now.

When we arrived back at St. Agatha's we found that the
75th B.G.H. was on the move again. To our dismay, we learned
that we were to go under canvas. It was March. The weather
was cold, wet and windy and the earth still hard from winter
but all that brand-new camping gear bought in Edinburgh had
to be tried out. The site was the football field attached to a large
psychiatric hospital in the environs of Birmingham. After many
shivering nights, we eventually achieved the knack of keeping
warm, clean and in good order in a confined space, irrespective
of the weather.

The only piece of camping equipment literally to let us down
was the collapsible bath. This was not well designed and we
could not make it work efficiently. After a fair trial which ended
each time with our sitting on a muddy tent floor with very cold
bottoms, we ditched it. Our greatest comfort was the Beatrice
paraffin stove. We each had one and with its mica window glow-
ing red and coffee heating on the top, it brought us warmth and
cheer on the coldest night.

By April, we were quite at home in our patched old bell tents
and the first sunny days found us catching up with arrears of
washing. A figure came hurrying from the hospital with the
morning post.

'Will you *listen*, everybody!' It was Janet Smart with her

chiming Scottish voice that did not carry very well. 'We're leaving at 1400 hrs *today*!'

We had no idea where we were going as we piled into the back of a three-ton truck at 1400 hrs precisely and set off due south by the sun. There were no clues during the long ride, for place names had been erased from signposts under the threat of invasion. We rattled through anonymous villages and came to rest in the early evening outside The Lamb public house in a village which turned out to be Angmering in Sussex.

Smithy, the Company Officer, dapper as a tin soldier, sprang from the back of a Utility vehicle and set about organising billets for the unit. Updown Cottage, an empty and sadly neglected little house next to the butcher's shop, could sleep eight so Pin, Duff, Soutie and I moved in quickly and bagged the downstairs room.

Angmering had played host to Poles and Canadians as well as British troops over the last few months and the cottage had been occupied by a series of military personnel but we were the first women. Mr. Cummings, the butcher, beamed his approval and slipped us a gin and tonic each as we moved in next door.

With makeshift curtains at the windows, we set up our campbeds in unaccustomed comfort. We had a roof over our heads and electric light at the end of a switch. Soutie, her ear to the ground as usual, reported . . . 'Staff Sergeant Regardsoe says we're here for a last kit issue and then we're off.'

The nature of the kit would tell us a lot. You did not get tropical kit for Norway nor duffle coats for southern Italy.

'Then what?'

Duff reached for an eyebrow pencil. She pointed to the wall above the fireplace. 'To join that lot, wherever they're going.'

Chalked on the wall in scrawling letters were the names of the previous occupants of the cottage.

East Yorks.

King's Shropshire Light Infantry.

Royal Winnipeg Rifles.

Underneath them, Duff added us. Q.A.I.M.N.S/R. of the 75th B.G.H. 'There,' she said. 'We're in good company.'

The kit issue, when it came a few days later, was depressing. It consisted simply of regulation men's khaki battledress trousers and jacket but treated with chemicals to repel vermin, particularly body lice. We were similarly unattracted to the material which resembled hairy cardboard and was no more comfortable to wear. In addition, the outfit had been designed for men. The unyielding trousers were too tight over the behind, too big around the waist and too long in the leg except for giraffes like Miss Agate. All of us, and especially the Matron, Miss Davies, who did not fancy herself even in well-cut slacks, were in despair as we carried away our new wardrobe from the church hall where the Q.M. had set up shop. It was time someone informed the War Office of the differences between men and women.

In addition to the anti-vermin outfit – A.V.s, as they came to be called – there were heavy, brown boots with soles like crumpets, and webbing to fasten around the ankle. There was a groundsheet which doubled as a rain cape, a protective outer garment of gas-proof material, a haversack containing a respirator, and a waterbottle, all of which had to be carried on the person. To someone like me, only five foot tall, this costume spelt total immobility.

Mr. Cummings, the butcher, found us trying on our new uniforms. Margaret Anderson was standing in barrel-like trousers which fitted her hips but left enough room at the waist for another Q.A. 'I'll fetch the wife,' he spluttered as he rushed off.

Mrs. Cummings was a tower of strength. With the aid of the Women's Institute Sewing Circle, the Sock Group and the Balaclava Bee, she converted our A.V.s from fancy dress into a wearable uniform. To complete our military appearance, we were given flashes to be sewn on the sleeve, and amongst them was the red and blue badge of 21st Army Group. When the dreaded, full-dress rehearsal came, in public, outside The Lamb we looked almost soldierly, except for the burgeoning breast pockets and something aggressive about the seat of the pants. R.S.M. Regan knew when he was beaten and gave up.

From then on, we wore A.V.s all the time and there was to be only one more airing for our grey and scarlet walking-out suits. The occasion was a Services dance at the nearby coastal town of Littlehampton on a fine evening at the beginning of June. It was hot on the crowded dance floor and several of us went up to the flat roof to cool off after the exertions of the Palais Glide. It was a still evening. The sea below us quietly lapped the deserted beach. Then above the muffled beat of the fox-trot came a new noise, a scarcely perceptible vibration at first that grew louder with every passing minute.

'Look!' Someone cried out in amazement and we watched a cloud of tiny specks in the sky behind us, fanning out and multiplying, as formation after formation of planes rose from the land and thundered overhead on their way out to sea. The noise was deafening now, bringing the dancers up from the ballroom floor below and the townsfolk out into the streets, moon-faces turned up to the sky.

Lancasters, Blenheims, and Halifaxes towing gliders, moved purposefully across the sky and headed for the coast of France. Like the 'Ah-ah-h-h' that follows a firework display, a great sigh went up from all of us who were watching, as we realised we were witnessing the opening of the Second Front.

It was a moment of elation and awe, 5th June, 1944.

There was no more dancing at Littlehampton that night. We returned soberly to Updown Cottage and found the whole village awake and wondering. The next morning, the B.B.C. gave out the great news that the Allies had landed in Normandy. We spent the day listening for every scrap of news over the wire-less.

At the end of that first day, the Allies had a toe-hold in Europe, in some places no more than a mile deep. Americans, British, Poles and Canadians were all there at different points of the thirty mile stretch involved, but not all of them had been able to make contact with each other. There were heavily forti-fied German positions between the Americans and the British, the British and the Canadians. The important bridges over the

Caen canal and the River Orne, which had been number one
target for the 6th Airborne Division on landing the night before,
were not taken until the evening of D-Day, after very heavy
fighting, when seaborne troops were able to relieve the hard-
pressed paratroopers. Tanks, men, transports and supplies
were now needed with the utmost speed, and for this the co-
operation of the English Channel – a notoriously untrustworthy
ally – was essential. Calm seas and fine weather were vital now
for the necessary build-up.

Our departure from Angmering and from our good friends,
Mr. and Mrs. Cummings, came a week later. We locked up the
cottage and took the key next door. The regiments who had
autographed the wall were even then carving themselves a bit
of glory. The East Yorks had dashed ahead at La Rivière,
silenced the fire from a massive pill-box, and went on to fight for
every yard of the town. King's Shropshire Light Infantry were
going it alone on the way to Caen because their supporting units
had failed to materialise, and the Royal Winnipeg Rifles were
attacking the River Seulles defences.

'I'll write,' promised Mrs. Cummings, and she did. Little
parcels of coffee, biscuits and hand-knitted socks to wear under
our gumboots were to seek us out wherever we went.

'Don't do anything I wouldn't do!' beamed the butcher, wiping his hands on his striped apron before seeing us to the door of
his shop, customers nodding and smiling.

Our hospital convoy now set off on a mystery tour, doubling
back, turning in circles until we had lost all sense of direction.
We had no idea where we were when our truck eventually
stopped, deep in a dense forest, and deposited us outside a
strongly guarded enclosure. The rest of the unit continued to
another site. It was women only here.

Grim-faced soldiers with tommy guns barred our entrance
into this secret marshalling camp until every identity card had
been scrutinised, then we were led under the umbrella of trees to
a carefully camouflaged administration hut staffed by serious-
minded A.T.S. officers. They doled out strange gifts, a tin of
concentrated meat each and a bar of chocolate to be tucked

away for emergencies, a container of water-purifying tablets, a French phrase book and a packet of French francs.

Supper, they told us soberly, as if they were convinced it would be our last, would be served in the dining hut within half an hour. Reveille at 0700 hours.

We were going to France but not to the site originally planned for us on the plain near Caen, for that city, which had been a D-Day objective, was still in German hands twelve days later because of the unexpected concentration of first class German troops in the area. A new site would have to be found for the 75th, probably in conjunction with the 81st B.H.G. which had just sailed. There was, as yet, little enough liberated country for the setting up of hospitals on a beachhead which was no more than twenty miles at its deepest penetration and only six miles at its weakest.

We left the marshalling camp the next morning and rejoined the rest of the unit, Duff, Pin, Soutie and I all in the same truck. It was 19th June. Long lines of transports were making for the docks at Southampton and we found ourselves in a stream of tanks and jeeps, of British, Canadian, American, Free French and Polish troops, cheered on our way by the entire population of the city. There was a sort of hysteria in the streets that day, with everyone laughing and clowning as if it was a carnival parade.

As women, we came in for special treatment. Our truck was flanked by a self-appointed escort of the crack Polish Motor-Cycle Brigade and collected special salutes from the policemen on point duty. American G.I.s, edging by in their jeeps, threw chocolate and tins of grapefruit into the back of our truck.

'Come and hold my hand, Nursie!' they yelled, and the crowd roared approvingly, waving them on their way to untimely death and mutilation.

Down on the bleak quay, the sky turned ominous. The festival atmosphere was missing. Drab, grey ships slewed with the turning tide; the restless water slapped and ran, and there was a hint of rain in the wind. We took our place amongst the troops, guns and transports waiting there and speculated on which of the ships was ours.

The Captain of the *Invicta*, a peace-time cross-Channel ferry, regarded our unit unenthusiastically from the bridge and gave the order to embark. Our C.O. hurried over to the Matron. 'Suggest we get your ladies on board first,' he said, with a meaningful glance at the wolf-whistling troops.

'Whenever you say, Colonel.' The Matron was hating this public exhibition, longing to embark. She led the way with a firm step. The crown on her shoulder precluded any comment from the troops but they had lost any reverence by the time I came along. I was last in the line, almost obliterated by my equipment. At every step, the tin mug at my waist clanked against the water-bottle and my rolled-up groundsheet poked my tin hat over my eyes. I tried not to waggle my bottom as I marched past the G.I.s but I was greeted with a roar of delight.

'Get off your knees, Shortie!'

'Why don't you get outa that hole, Lootenant?'

With flaming face, I clumped angrily up the gangway behind Duff, who somehow managed to look willowy, even in this outfit.

There were not enough cabins for fifty women as well as the medical officers so we would have to make do with hammocks amidships on the Mess-deck, an ill-lit area next to the galley that smelt of stale cabbage. There were no portholes. We peered unenthusiastically into the gloom. Trestle tables. Wooden benches. It looked most unpromising.

'Now then,' a party of A.B.s, very jolly, came clattering down the companionway. 'We're going to show you 'ow to sling a 'ammock.'

And then they had to show us how to get in, fully dressed, boots and all, for that was the order of dress for the voyage. It was only for one night, we consoled ourselves, and went up on deck to see the last of England.

We had no sooner left the protection of the coast, than the *Invicta* started to wallow in a most unpleasant swell. The First Officer, pointing to the banks of clouds that were building up, reminded us that the day was D-13. A strengthening wind tipped the waves with white and soon there was a Force Nine gale blowing. The 'fiddles' went up round the tables and the deck took on outlandish angles, shipping an occasional swathe of green water. Jokes about seasickness died away as we swallowed our pills and tried to put out of our minds that splendid American breakfast of pancakes and maple syrup, bacon and eggs.

In all, we took three and a half days to cross the little stretch of water that separated us from France. Unable to put back into port for security reasons, we zig-zagged about, to and fro, under the lee of the land. We were short of bread and of water. The galley was a shambles and unable to produce hot meals, not that many of us could have eaten them anyway, for we were all very seasick. Nights on the stuffy Mess-deck were miserable as we swung, netted and trussed up, still in our uncomfortable uniform. Only ankle webbing was allowed to be removed in a concession towards comfort. We cursed the jaunty sailor on the Tannoy with his 'Wakey! Wakey!' every morning. We struggled out of the encapsulating hammocks to clatter, still banana-shaped, on to the tables underneath that were already being laid with basins of cold porridge and slabs of corned beef by hardbitten sailors who had seen it all before. This, and the smell from the galley, was usually enough to send us running to the heaving 'heads'.

'Fresh air is what you need.' Capt. Johnson, the dental officer, marched us, green-faced, around the swilling deck. In addition to feeling sick, we became chilled to the marrow and half-drowned.

We were unable to see the funny side as Lt. Colonel Murray, i/c Medical Division and fitness fanatic, staggered his self-imposed daily mile around the deck, baring his teeth at the storm in a stoical grin and singing, when he could find the breath, snatches from 'A Life on the Ocean Wave'. Nothing was amusing any more. What really kept us going was the lifesaving two ounce measure of overproof rum ordered by the Captain for everyone on board.

This freakish storm put the whole ambitious invasion plan in jeopardy and threatened the Allies with disaster. Out-going

convoys were driven back time and time again and mines trig-
gered off by the force of the storm sank more ships that way
than on D-Day itself. The fate of the whole enterprise hung in
the balance for three days.

Gradually, the storm abated. The galley no longer rang with
the crashing of broken pots. At last, we felt sufficiently recovered
to toy with a water biscuit and hot Bovril, and were relieved
beyond measure by the sighting of a smudge on the horizon.
We were looking at the coast of France. The arms of the
Mulberry harbour at Arromanches reached out to us. The
Invicta slipped inside and dropped anchor.

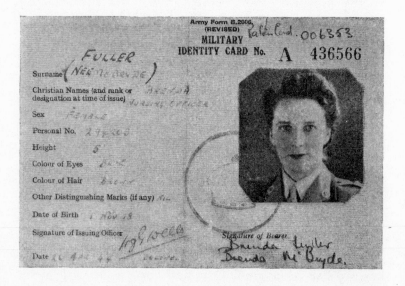

6

In Normandy with the 81st B.G.H.

The land rose gently in dunes from a beach still littered with the debris of the landing seventeen days earlier. Burnt-out tanks had settled into the pale sand, blown-up trucks lay abandoned on their backs. An amphibious craft, wrecked before it reached the shore, poked its grey snout from the shallows. There were jerrycans everywhere and torn clothing fluttered from barbed wire defences. Over the whole of the land, as far as we could see, hung a pall of smoke. This was not the France of Colette or Chevalier that I had hoped some day to visit but a France under German occupation where, before long, every village would become a battlefield. As we crowded the ship's rails, two planes circled in combat high above us.

The need ashore for supplies and men was urgent. For the last three days, only a quarter of the expected ammunition and guns had been able to land because of the storm. Two and a half miles of prefabricated roadway had been sent to the bottom of the sea within sight of France. Hitler could not have engineered a better ally than that three-day gale so soon after D-Day.

Figures now appeared on the beach, hurrying towards the M.T.B.s tied up there. There was a sound of engines turning over and two launches came spanking across the harbour towards us in a half-circle of spray and drew alongside the *Invicta*. An A.B. pushed through us to the rails, his arms full of rope ladder, the significance of which filled us with dismay, and from the launch below, a young naval lieutenant looked up into our mistrustful faces.

'Let's be having you,' he called up lightheartedly, as if one clambered down a rope ladder every day of one's life 'And don't fall in, for I may not be brave enough to go in after you.'

Annie P. Scott from County Cork was at the head of the line

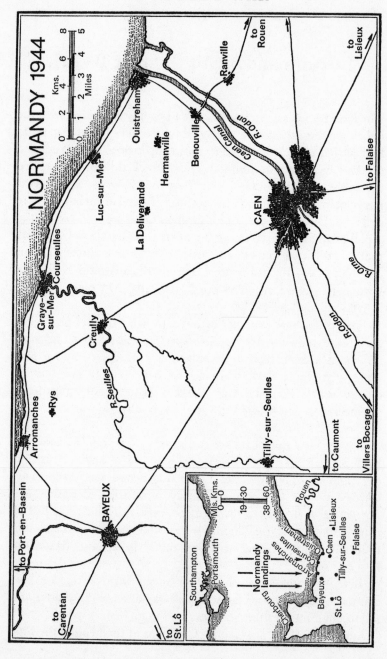

NORMANDY 1944

Kms.
Miles

to Rouen
to Lisieux
Ranville
Ouistreham
Hermanville
Benouville
Caen Canal
R. Odon
Luc-sur-Mer
La Deliverande
CAEN
to Falaise
Graye-sur-Mer Courseulles
Creully
R. Orne
R. Odon
R. Seulles
Rys
Tilly-sur-Seulles
to Caumont
Arromanches
to Villers Bocage
to Port-en-Bassin
BAYEUX
to Carentan
to St. Lô

Mls. Kms.
Rouen
Southampton
Portsmouth
Cherbourg
Arromanches
Ouistreham
Courseulles
Caen • Lisieux
Tilly-sur-Seulles
Falaise
Normandy landings
Bayeux
St.Lô

'Spoken like a true English gentleman,' she said bitterly as she grabbed the rope and gingerly swung over one leg.

'Sure, I'm a brave Irishman like yourself, darlin',' and he gave the rope a playful tug that brought Annie's eyes out on stalks.

Behind us, the crew of the *Invicta* were already hosing down the decks as if to be rid of a nasty contagion, and the men of our unit were filling the other launch. There was nothing for it but to grit one's teeth and go over the side with the best face possible. I looked apprehensively at the choppy grey water as I took my turn at the rail. If I fell in, I hadn't a hope of keeping afloat with all this gear on.

Margaret Anderson was the last to go over. We watched her now from the safety of the launch as, with white face and tight lips, she thrust one leg over the side and fumbled for the rope. But she was hampered by the water-bottle at her waist and the bulky field dressing in its knee pocket. She missed her footing on the rung and, clutching the rope desperately to her chest, she began to swing alarmingly, now over the water, now over our anxious heads.

'Jesus and Mary, Mother of God,' breathed Scott devoutly, 'she's going in the drink.'

However, Andy's scrabbling feet found a rung and she began to descend. Willing hands stretched out to help her as she slid the last yard into the arms of a, by now, thoroughly frightened young officer. His voice shook. 'Welcome aboard, Ma'am.'

The launch carrying the men had already left the ship and was making for the shore, but we were deposited with our gear on one arm of the artificial harbour, still some distance from the land. Transport, the lieutenant told us, was on its way to collect us and, with that, he returned to the *Invicta* to pick up the rest of the men. We watched from the breakwater while the remainder of the unit splashed ashore from the launches, formed up on the beach then plunged over the sandy dunes to be lost from sight.

The *Invicta* pulled up anchor and steamed away to pick up

wounded from a point further along the coast, leaving a suddenly empty sea around us. Splintered ammunition boxes and empty food tins bumped against the piers at our feet and a light rain began to fall. We wrapped ourselves in groundsheets and searched the coastline for signs of the promised transport.

Small fires were beginning to prick the darkening dunes as men who were dug in there set about preparing their evening meal. The sky to the east took on an angry flush. This distant area pulsating with gunfire was Caen, where we should have been setting up our hospital. As it was, we were to join the 81st B.G.H. who, because of the storms, had been left to cope with the bulk of the casualties in this congested area for the last three days.

Eventually our transport came, two trucks well marked with red crosses. As we clattered over metal treads laid across the beach, men of the Survey Regiment, who had been living in the dunes since D-Day, emerged from their foxholes with disbelief on their faces. 'White women!' they yelled, and crowded around the open backs of the trucks; men in string vests and berets. They wore whatever was convenient for living in a hole in the sand.

'How's London and the Flying Bombs?'

'Got any bread?'

'Got any papers?' But our newspapers were four days old.

'Four days! Which way did you come? Round the Cape?'

From the beach, we followed the route taken by 50 (Northumbrian) Division on D-Day, a road intended for farm carts which was now breaking up under the traffic of troops and heavy armour. Military directions and unit identifications crowded the verges, along with the sinister black skull and crossbones of the German mine warning: 'Achtung! Minen!'

'I lof you,' a little boy called out from the top of a farmhouse gate. 'Chewing gomme? Ceegarettes?' but his mother called him away and did not return our friendly wave. These quiet Normandy farms had borne the brunt of our naval bombardment and the few French people we saw moved dispiritedly about their damaged homes and were not inclined to make any gesture of welcome towards us. Who would replace the dead cattle? Who would build the new barn and repair the broken fences? The orchards we passed by were pocked with shell craters and the poplars were stripped by blast. France was everybody's battlefield.

'They don't seem very pleased to see us,' murmured Duff, beside me at the open end of the truck. 'Can't blame them, I suppose. Look at the holes in their roofs.'

We found the 81st B.G.H. near the little village of Rys in a field by the main road. A convoy of ambulances coming from the opposite direction followed us through the entrance gates on a rubble road past the tented wards to the reception area. Even in the fading light, we could recognise the standard lay-out of a field hospital, the one-way route flanked by marquee tents of the surgical wards and crossed at right angles by roads sign-posted to the Pathology Department, Dental Department and X-ray. At the heart of the encampment was the parking bay for ambulances and the Reception tent where all casualties were seen on arrival. Close at hand were the Hospital Office, the C.O.'s office and the Quartermaster's Store. Cookhouse and unit personnel tents were pitched some distance away.

The men from our unit had marched here and were already settled in. As we climbed down from the trucks, we could see our own Colonel in earnest conversation with the 81st Staff Officers in their Hospital Office. Ambulances with 'Casualty' boards swinging from their radiators were still coming in from the road and lining up alongside us. Suddenly, we were in the centre of a whirl of activity as M.O.'s came to attend to the new arrivals and clerks hurried to and from the Hospital Office with sheaves of papers in their hands. As our Matron went off to confer with the C.O., stretcher-bearers plodded by on their way to the wards with their burden of grey-faced men, men with eyes closed and bloodied field dressings about their heads, men in the act of being transfused, an orderly walking alongside with bottle of blood held high. A tense sister with a towel pinned over her battledress whipped by without a sideways glance. Everyone, it seemed, had a job to do but us.

As we waited, searchlights began to sweep the sky and the night suddenly cracked open with a bombardment that made us jump. The ack-ack guns must surely be in the next field, but the clerks hurrying by seemed to accept it all as a regular performance.

On the way to the marquee that had been set aside for us, we had to pass the wards, blazing with bare light, their canvas sides a shadow-play of feverish activity, figures stooping, hands lifting, heads bending. As the stretcher bearers tunnelled head-down through the entrance flaps, we were given a shocking glimpse of what was going on inside, wounded men packed so tightly that there was hardly room for the two harassed sisters to move. We could hear the low moans of the injured, feel the tension and the trauma in there. How could we stand aside? But our Matron urged us firmly on.

'Not tonight. We relieve the 81st tomorrow morning. Find your kit now and get some sleep.' She went off with the Assistant Matron and we were left to locate our bedrolls from a heap piled high on the grass. There was a biscuit tin of hot water for each of us behind a strip of hessian, and we were able to have the first decent wash since leaving England. It was sheer bliss to peel off rumpled girdles and wash all over, to stand with bare feet in the tin full of water after wearing laced boots for four days.

Before our two overworked batmen went off duty, they left us self-heating tins of cocoa, plates of corned beef, ships' biscuits and a piece of advice. 'Sleep with your tin hats over the place where you wouldn't like to have an operation.' They looked thoughtfully skywards where the barrage was continuing relentlessly. 'What goes up must come down.'

In spite of the racket, we prepared for bed. People fussed about, getting comfortable for the night; Janet Smart with her mug of cold water in case she was thirsty in the 'wee sma' hours', tucked away in a corner beside Andy, her inseparable companion, who was already ceremoniously laid out for sleep, flat on her back, legs straight, arms by her side, her tin hat balanced exactly on her nose; the Irish contingent in a giggling group, the pair from the Shetlands, quietly communing. Inside my bed-roll, I rubbed one clean bare foot sensually against the other, old friends, happy to meet up again. As I adjusted my tin hat, I noticed that Duff, alongside me, had different priorities. She was lying on her stomach with her tin hat over her bottom. We were all so thankful to be able to lie horizontally on firm ground that did not pitch, toss or roll, that we forgot about the barrage and slept deeply right through the night.

The batman, Sharatt, had some difficulty in waking us the next morning. His violent bashing on a biscuit tin eventually penetrated my consciousness and, opening my eyes, I stared at the tent top. I could not, at first, remember where I was. There were none of the creaking, swishing noises of days at sea but the sound of birds and the crunch of boots on clinker. Then I remembered we were in Normandy.

Around me, the tent was in a shambles. Gear was everywhere and crumpled A.V.s hung from the tentpoles like dejected old men. Boots and water-bottles were kicked about. There was a smell of roots, and mushrooms, and dirty socks. Pin, in pyjamas, was bending over a steaming dixie at the tent door.

'Tea up.'

Figures began to emerge from bedrolls, oddly unfamiliar in the strange, almost submarine, green light reflected from the grass that was our carpet. Soutie, her face in shadow, was struggling to pull on gumboots, bound for the ablutions at the top of the field. I stepped into my A.V.s with distaste. We were to go on duty in the wards this morning. This was our first nursing since Peebles and it was in another world. I had worn a crisp cotton uniform then, with a white head veil. I hunted now in my kit for a clean shirt, and put scissors, fountain pen and a handful of safety pins into the breast pocket. It seemed a modest preparation for a day of God knows what.

We breakfasted off tinned bacon and the inevitable ships' biscuits, then made for the Matron's tent to learn the order of duty. Some of us were required to work only until midday so that we could get some sleep before going on duty that night. The rest of us were detailed off in pairs to relieve the 81st sisters on each ward. I was to work with Audrey Dare, a solidly practical girl with the staying power of an ox, and we set off together for the Resuscitation department, past incinerators gobbling rubbish and field boilers spluttering with hot water. The night's bombardment had stopped with the coming of the daylight, and distant guns sounded no more lethal than summer thunder.

The Resuscitation department formed one arm of a U-shaped arrangement of tents with the theatre as a bridge leading to a surgical ward. It was floored with a heavy tarpaulin ground-sheet and stacked with trestles to support the stretchers of wounded as they arrived from the ambulances. Here the men were given intensive treatment for shock until they were sufficiently restored to undergo operation, after which they passed straight from the theatre to the wards.

At the entrance to Resus., was the treatment area, a table covered by a sheet on which were laid trays of instruments, syringes, sterilisers etc., had been laid out. Upended wooden boxes provided shelves for medicines and dressings; splints were stacked in a clean dustbin, and large, wooden chests contained the transfusion apparatus. On the other side of the entrance was a makeshift desk which bore the Admission Book and an array of requisition forms for diets, dispensary, replacements and repairs, extra blankets, pillows.

Thirty casualties had been admitted into Resus., during the night, all but two of whom had now been operated on and transferred to the adjoining ward. The two sisters from the 81st who were going off duty now handed over these remaining casualties, and wearily made for breakfast and bed, leaving Audrey and me in charge.

The two men lying so still on their stretchers with eyes closed were from the 7th Armoured Division. Both had been badly wounded in an abortive attempt to take an enemy pillbox. They had lost a great deal of blood but were now beginning to respond to the transfusions which had gone on all night. We were registering their blood pressures when one of our own surgeons from the 75th, Major MacPherson, a Canadian, came in.

He raised sandy eyebrows towards us. 'You settled in all right?' He felt under the grey blankets of one of the stretchers for a pulse and bent down close to the soldiers's pale face. 'We'll get you to the theatre presently, son. Fix up that leg. OK?'

The soldier, who had a huge gunshot wound of thigh, made an almost imperceptible movement of his eyelids. He was swinging between reality and unconsciousness. We went to the desk to check his transfusion chart.

'Give him saline next and we'll do him first on the list.' Major MacPherson sighed and lowered his voice. 'I'm not looking forward to operating in that tent.'

With Sister Agate in charge, he would not even notice that the theatre was a tent.

'Sir,' George Easton, the Resuscitation orderly attached to the 81st, stood at the tent entrance. We turned at the urgency in his voice. 'Convoy of wounded on the way.'

'Inform Lt. Colonel Harding, i/c 75th Surgical Division,' Major MacPherson said sharply and went to the door as a string of ambulances went by on their way to Reception.

The taking of Tilly-sur-Seulles on 18th June had been a great victory for XXX Corps. Now, five days later, they were meeting stiff resistance in the high ground south of Tilly. This battle was being translated to us in a grim toll of casualties.

We entered the names of many famous regiments into the Admission Book that day: the Staffordshire Yeomanry, 4th Wilts, Dorsets, Green Howards, and East Yorks, men of the 7th Armoured Division and 50 (Northumbrian) Division. Most of their proud uniform, stiff with blood and caked in mud, had to be cut from them. We sliced the tough boots with razors to release shattered feet. The stretcher bearers came again and again until every trestle was occupied and the floor crammed so that there was barely room to put a foot or kneel between the stretchers. Audrey and I accompanied Lt. Colonel Harding and Major MacPherson as they went from one man to the next, assessing his condition and setting up transfusions.

In the trauma of that first day, everything I had learnt during four hard years of training suddenly made sense. My hands had a sure and certain skill and my brain was unflustered as I replaced dressings over gaping wounds, gave injections of morphia and the new wonder drug, penicillin, charted blood pressures. I began to see, for the first time, that the disciplines of the training school were a necessary part of the whole. That tent, full of men, reeking of blood, was where I was needed. These men, whose clammy bodies overpowered me with the nauseous sweet smell of shock were my fulfilment, since they could no longer help themselves.

Down on my knees, I swabbed a vein for Major MacPherson, ready with the transfusion canula, and the soldier, deep in shock, sighed profoundly, searching for air as he stared in an unrelated way at the bottle of red blood hanging over him. Stepping over splinted limbs and stretcher handles, we moved to the next man, a penetrating wound of chest, needing a large firm dressing to contain those ominous sucking noises and another pillow to keep him upright.

Lt. Colonel Harding, one stretcher ahead with Audrey Dare, kept up a running commentary. 'Stomach here. Put him number one. Quarter of morphia, Sister. Straight away. Two pints of blood, one of plasma ...' Gunshot, mortar blast, mines, incendiaries. Limbs, eyes, abdomen, chest. He chewed his pencil. Who had priority? Of all these desperately wounded men, whose need was the most urgent?

We came at last to the end of the casualty intake and the two surgeons left for the operating theatre, leaving Audrey and me to carry out resuscitation treatment. Penicillin, in those early days, was given in massive doses of 3000 units by three-hourly injections and it seemed to us that we had no sooner completed one round when the next was due. We found that we had in George Easton a solid, reliable orderly. With written instructions in one hand, he moved delicately among the injured men with his bucket of 'Compo' tea, helping those who were permitted a drink.

This Compo tea took some getting used to. It came in the form of a cube, a dehydrated amalgam of tea, sugar and milk, and was simplicity itself to make. There was none of the mystique of warming the pot and covering with a cosy. With Compo tea, you merely threw a handful of cubes into a bucket and poured on boiling water to the desired level, gave it a stir, and there it was. Crude, perhaps, but wonderfully fortifying and, before the summer was out, we were drinking it by the gallon.

Left to his own pace, Easton worked well and with great thoughtfulness, but an unthinking, sharp word from Audrey or myself could wreck his composure and confidence. We had to learn to keep haste out of our voices and remember that, after all, he was not a nurse, but a farm labourer with the patience of Job. He was continually amazed and humbled that these brave fighting men needed his help, and he was as gentle with them as a mother with her child. He had handled baby lambs and other small animals for most of his life and his big hands were never rough or clumsy.

He mothered us, too. That first morning, the hours flew by unheeded, and it was Easton who brought us a plate of cheese and biscuits and a basin of tea when it was long past noon. It would have been impossible for either of us to leave the ward to go to the Mess and he had privately decided to get us some lunch.

'It's only French stuff,' he apologised. 'No Cheddar or anything.'

We sat on a blood box and ate a superb, ripe Camembert and drank sweet tea from half-pint tin basins, speaking quietly together in case we might fail to hear any more urgent sound than the gentle, sighing 'Oh dear's' whispering around the canvas. Men brought to Resus. were always in a serious condition, some of them *in extremis*, past meaningful speech or any sustained communication. Each man was an island in his own desperation, unaware of other men on other stretchers, but their utterances were all the same. There were no impassioned calls to God, no harking back to mother, only an infinitely sad 'Oh dear', from colonels and corporals alike.

That was our first morning. After that, we knew what it was all about. Some time during that day, a familiar name leapt at me from a soldier's record card. These were the medical notes contained in a waterproof envelope which was tied to a button on the man's battledress by the first M.O. to see him, usually at a Regimental Aid Post or Field Dressing Station. As I skimmed through the notes, I would have recognized the terrible hand-writing even without the signature at the bottom – S. Raw. Major. R.A.M.C. Our beloved registrar from the Newcastle hospital was not too far away and I wondered how many more friends were around.

Gradually, as the day wore on, spaces were cleared between the stretchers as the wounded were sent for operation and then passed through to the wards. Soutie, Pin and Duff were working at that end, getting the men we had resuscitated straight from the theatre, to be watched and nursed with care. There could be nothing static about the occupants of the wards, however. Our Normandy bridgehead was too small for the accumulation of casualties and they must be evacuated by sea or air as soon as they were fit to travel. On that first day, the 81st Company Officer went the rounds of the wards with our own Lt. Smith and a scribbling clerk, preparing an evacuation list for the next day.

Those who died were given a simple burial service by the hospital padre. The areas set aside for them, marked with simple white wooden crosses, have become the well-tended military cemeteries of today.

It was especially important for us in Resus. to keep the casualties moving since, in every convoy, the majority of the wounded needed to come to us for shock treatment. With each man dispatched to the theatre, there was a trestle cleared for the next convoy and no-one knew when that might arrive.

The 75th theatre team settled quickly into the new routine and by the middle of the afternoon it was as if they had never operated under any other conditions. Amputations, burns, abdominals: it would have been a daunting list even for a civilian theatre. As far as Miss Agate was concerned, it was just another field hospital. It took a great deal to remove that con-fident smile from her composed features. In addition, the

O.R.A.s, orderlies trained as operating room assistants, knew their job backwards. Correct glove sizes, full drums of sterile towels and dressings, transfusion apparatus; the equipment was always ready at hand, the sucker machine in working order. Everything was there, even in a tent. Over a lightweight operating table hung a powerful lamp that was run off the dynamo in the field outside. There was a scrubbing-up annexe stacked with jerrycans of water and enamel basins, equipped by Pioneers with an adequate soakaway. Conditions were as aseptic as it was possible to achieve.

All day long and for most of the night too, heaps of dirty instruments descended on the back-shop orderly to be scrubbed, sterilised and put back into service. The surgeons saw little of that fine, June day and the linen bins overflowed with their discarded gowns.

The next convoy arrived around six o'clock that evening. Our Resus. tent was filled to the doors again. When blood pressures and pulses had to be charted every fifteen minutes, penicillin and morphia given and wounds redressed, Audrey and I had no time for anything more than a passing word.

Easton went by with his arms full of tattered uniforms. The pile on the tarpaulin had been growing all day as we cut the cloth from wounds. 'I'll take this lot to the incinerator, Sister.' Hard-won stripes and pips and crowns, sewn on by proud Mums, wives and girl friends: the leaping black boar of XXX Corps, the blue and red flash of 21 Army group. It was all the same now. The field incinerator smoked all night.

7

At the Front Line: Hermanville

Three days later, on 26th June, any sisters of the 75th B.G.H. who could be spared from the 81st were detailed to help at certain points east of Rys where there was difficulty in evacuating the wounded. Sustained and accurate shelling by the Germans of landing strips and beaches in the area near Caen was not only preventing the landing of supplies, which was the enemy's intention, but was creating a serious bottleneck of casualties. Hotels at Graye-sur-Mer, Luc-sur-Mer and Courseulles were full of wounded men awaiting evacuation to England. Several of our sisters, including Pin, Duff and Soutie, were posted to help at these points while I, with Audrey Dare, Barbara Burr and Joan Deadman, was sent to the aid of a Field Dressing Station six miles north-west of Caen, near the village of Hermanville.

The function of a Field Dressing Station, which was always in a forward position, was to resuscitate, operate and evacuate. There were no sisters on the unit strength since it was not designed to hold casualties. Now, with evacuation almost brought to a standstill, the C.O., Major Edwards, had a tent full of men needing post-operative care. We were going in answer to his urgent request for trained nurses.

It was now three weeks since the Allied landing and the bridgehead was still no deeper than twenty miles at its greatest penetration near Caumont and measured less than eight miles in the Caen sector. The dramatic reduction in the supply of guns and men brought about by the storm had seriously slowed down our advances. Caen was still strongly held by the Germans and, on our right flank, the American drive had ground to a halt in front of the heavily defended St. Lô area although they had made great gains in the Cotentin peninsula and the port of Cherbourg was on the point of surrender. In spite of Herculean efforts on the part of the French Resistance to delay the arrival of German reinforcements from the south of France, these were now lining up in formidable strength in the Caen area and in the strategically important heights south of Tilly, blocking the way across the rivers Odon and Orne.

With the beach-head thus tentatively held, the weather brought further complications as rain began to fall steadily, turning the lanes and fields into quagmires. On the morning of our departure from Rys, men of the 49th Division were launching an attack on the River Odon and their perilous way was through flooded minefields under crossfire from enemy positions on the high ground. There would be rain-soaked and muddied casualties at the 81st before the day was out.

In gumboots and tin hats, and with groundsheets over our shoulders, Pin, Duff, Soutie and I sloshed through the rain to the waiting vehicles, an ambulance for the F.D.S. and a fifteen cwt. truck to take the others to the coast.

At an excited hail from behind, we turned to see Annie P. Scott towing a breathless padre.

'Come out, Margaret Fairy!' she called into the crowded truck. 'Come out and be blessed. I'll not see me little friend go into the Front Line without a drop of the Holy Water.' And while a Q.A. of her own faith emerged somewhat sheepishly from the truck, the padre was adjured to 'do his stuff'. With no great show of enthusiasm, which was not surprising considering the pouring rain, he rapidly made a few vague dispensations with a bottle of water while Annie beamed her approval, rain splashing down from her tin hat.

'Aye, and what about the Presbyterians?' came sharply from the interior of the truck. 'I suppose it doesna' matter what happens to us?'

We four who were bound for the F.D.S. squashed together in the front seat of the ambulance alongside the driver, determined to see as much of Normandy as we could. We had been working with the 81st B.G.H. for the last three days and this was the first opportunity to see the surrounding countryside. The fifteen cwt. truck carrying the other party made for the coast and we took the road to Creully, Caen and Hermanville. Rain sluiced down the windscreen, stotted off the radiator, streamed out of choked ditches and overflowed the shellholes. It was a desolate, waterlogged landscape and the few villages we passed through were scarred by shellfire. Black-shawled women moved among the remaining drab shops which seemed to sell nothing but coarse black bread and tortoiseshell combs. The surface of the road was badly broken up and we lurched alarmingly in and out of pot-holes. Burnt-out vehicles cluttered the verges. The jacket of some unfortunate farmer hung from a tree alongside his cart wheel over a mine warning he plainly had not seen.

At Creully we came upon a stream of refugee civilians fleeing with their possessions from Caen, a pall of smoke some twelve kilometres distant. Women and children and old men trudged in the rain, pushing handcarts and prams piled with pots and pans and bundles of clothing, seeking shelter with relatives and friends in more fortunate situations. They did not raise their eyes as we passed by.

Leaving the Caen road, we pressed on to Hermanville which had been taken on D-Day by the South Lancs. after bitter hand-to-hand fighting. It was now in ruins. The main street was broken up and heaped with rubble. Rain poured through the gaping roofs of empty cottages. Just past the church, which had miraculously escaped damage, we came to an encampment in a dripping orchard festooned with camouflage netting. There were Engineers here, a section of Field Artillery, a Searchlight battery and a squad of Pioneers. In a rain-soaked huddle of canvas near by was the F.D.S. we had come to join.

As we stepped down into the mud, a figure in streaming cape approached us and held out a welcoming hand. This was our new C.O., Major Edwards, looking as though he had not slept for a week.

'I expect you'd like a cup of coffee.' He led the way to the Mess.

The noise of gunfire was noticeably louder here for we were barely five miles from the front. The men lived in dug-outs roofed over with 'bivvy' tents. Predictably, our arrival caused a stir throughout the encampment. We were the first women the men had seen since leaving England and they had all been through a rough time. They crowded into the Mess tent, grinning all over their faces, to the embarrassment of Major Edwards. Obviously, this complication had not occurred to him when he sent in his request for sisters, but we hastened to assure him that we were quite able to look after ourselves.

He told us of the ward full of men needing a wash and a change of dressings and wearily ran a hand through his hair. 'My Number Two and I and the O.R.A.s have our hands full with the theatre and resuscitation. The ward is getting out of hand. That's why I asked for you.' He pushed back his chair. 'I'll show you the set-up then I'll flog my bunk for a spell.'

We pulled on our wet groundsheets once more and he hid a smile as we clapped on tin hats. 'There's something very bizarre about lipstick under a tin hat,' he said apologetically.

The F.D.S. tents comprised a resuscitation annexe leading to a theatre which opened on to the large ward tent. The whole outfit was dug in to a depth of about one and a half feet, and, no matter how hard the Pioneers drained the ground, persistent trickles of yellow water found their way under the canvas sides.

'This lousy weather,' cursed the Major as we slipped and slid down the entrance into the ward. Light from the doorway fell on the nearest stretchers where still figures lay, with eyes closed, like effigies in a churchyard. Reaching back into the shadows at the rear of the tent were trestles bearing horizontal shapes wrapped in grey blankets, with bottles of blood rearing over them like sinister crimson flowers on spindly stems. But the first impact was the smell, the smell of wounds needing to be dressed, the smell of sweat and the stink a man gets when his insides are giving up.

The Major apologised. 'Duncan is stretcher-bearer. He isn't trained for this sort of thing.'

We could see Duncan standing by a stretcher, feeding cup in one hand, urinal in the other, wrinkled trousers hoisted high on braces. He was a peacetime postman from Weston-Super-Mare who drove a little van and chatted up the housewives.

Major Edwards turned to us. 'Any problems?'

'If you can show us where we are to sleep,' said Audrey Dare very practically, 'two of us can get some rest before taking the night shift.'

The question of our sleeping quarters had already occupied the mind of the A.D.M.S. (Area Director Medical Services) and he had decided that the battlefront near Caen was too close for comfort. Arrangements had been made for us to sleep at a convent in the village of La Deliverande, a few miles back. We tossed for shifts and Audrey Dare and Barbara Burr took the night shift leaving immediately by ambulance with all our gear.

The Major handed us the keys to the drug cupboard. 'Keep all the drips going. There's an O.R.A. on duty in the theatre. He'll come for me if you need me.' He turned at the entrance. 'I hope you don't.'

He and his assistant surgeon had been getting no more than two hours sleep out of the twenty-four for the last week. We saw his bunk later. It was a muddy shelf dug into the side of a trench.

Joan Deadman and I rolled up our sleeves. There was no time to waste for the thought appalled us that more casualties might arrive before we could attend to the men already in the ward.

'Bucket of hot water, Duncan. Clean blankets, pyjamas, from any Q.M. you can find.'

Duncan hurried away, obviously relieved and we took stock of our patients. We began at the end of the line with a corporal of the 15th Scottish, half comatosed, with an uncertain grip on life. He had led an attack on a German gun position that was blocking the road ahead, taking the enemy by surprise with grenade and bayonet, and getting his own back for what the bastards had done on the Clyde. He'd silenced the gun but most of the lads he took with him had been silenced too. He, himself, was too badly wounded to move and had to lie there among the dead, awaiting stretcher-bearers. Later, Major Edwards repaired what he could of the torn blood vessels and muscles. At least, the corporal still had his leg.

Gently, we eased him out of his jacket and what was left of his trousers, still caked in mud from the hole where he had lain, and we rolled him on to his good side. There is not much room to manoeuvre on a stretcher and I cradled him firmly to me while Joan soaped and gently sponged his back, all reddened and pitted with bits of earth and grass. Then she rolled up the soiled blanket from underneath him and laid a clean one alongside. In this position, we drew on one sleeve of a pyjama jacket and rolled him smoothly over the hump of blankets to Joan. Swiftly now, because he was lying on his injured leg, I pulled away the dirty blanket, straightened in the clean one, eased on the rest of his pyjama jacket, then let him slip back gently on to a cool, clean pillow. With sterile towels pinned over our fronts, we renewed the dressing on his leg. It was a deep wound and would need skin replacement at a later date. I imagined him in the friendly ward at Bangour. Then we cleaned his furred tongue and crusted lips so that the sips of water that followed tasted sweet and good. We combed his dusty hair, charted temperature and blood pressure, gave him an injection of penicillin and left him to slide back into restorative sleep. It took forty minutes to make just one man comfortable.

The tank commander on the next trestle had learnt tank warfare in the Middle East, standing up, head and shoulders out of the turret as he surveyed the wide expanses of desert. Normandy was an entirely different terrain. The closely hedged lanes were ideal for enemy snipers and this reckless lieutenant had been shot at close range through the back. The bullets had penetrated one lung and narrowly missed his spine. Breathing was not easy for him. We stayed by him with the oxygen until his chest became more tranquil and his eyes less anxious.

Duncan worked hard, clearing away the soiled blankets as we whipped them out from under the men and reporting when any bottle of blood, plasma or saline became dangerously low. There were third degree burns to dress, chests to be aspirated of blood leaked there from a wound. The technique of the stump bandage learnt in the training school was a commonplace here amongst so many amputations.

At midday, we took a break, sitting on Compo boxes at the tent door where the air, if damper, was fresher. Huddled figures wrapped in groundsheets and carrying mess-tins appeared from time to time on their way to the dining tent, but we settled for a plate of Spam and mashed potato, and Duncan brought us half a bucket of tea from the cookhouse.

Our dress of shirt and trousers tucked into gumboots might seem odd for a hospital ward but it was right for the work we were doing. The tough, chemically treated cloth of our A.V.s was water-resistant and bore up well under all the kneeling on muddy tarpaulins that we had to do. When aseptic conditions were required, we scrubbed-up at a corner table and covered the whole of our fronts with a sterile towel. Our bare hands never touched a wound. Using instruments, we followed the 'no touch' technique all the time.

'Still three-quarters of the ward to do.' Joan's eyes were troubled. Her usually neat, dark hair which she wore in a roll around her head had become disarranged during the morning and escaping strands lay on the collar of her shirt. I knew I must look just as dishevelled.

'All right if we get no more casualties,' I said. But we did. In the middle of the afternoon, one of Major Edwards' orderlies came into the tent from the theatre.

'Casualties, Sister. Will you send Duncan to wake the Major?'

I went with him to the Resuscitation tent to await the M.O.s and found six or seven stretchers there, men from the 51st Highland Division who had been in a thrust to bypass Caen on the eastern side. They had come straight from their Regimental Aid Posts. Some were already being transfused, others would need it immediately. I prepared the transfusion sets, tourniquet, bottle of blood, drip stand, and by that time the Major, his assistant surgeon and anaesthetist were all there, looking as refreshed as if they had had twelve hours sleep instead of just over four. Next, there was bleeding to deal with, anti-tetanus injections to be given and anti-gas gangrene serum for the Jock who'd stepped on a mine. There was no hope of saving his leg

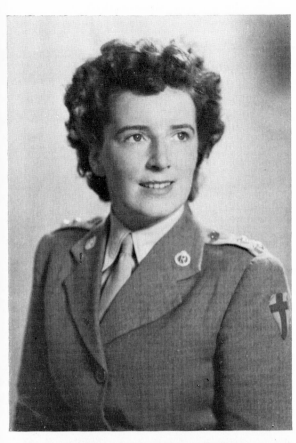

The author, 1943, in the grey and scarlet uniform of the Q.A.I.M.N.S/R.

Across the Rhine, after the German Retreat, May 1945

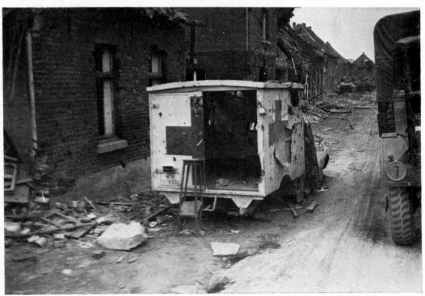

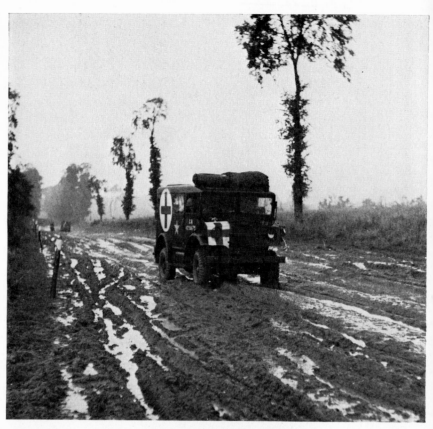

Red Cross ambulances driving through the mud in Normandy, July 1944

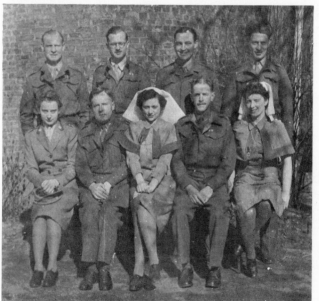

No. 5. Maxillo-Facial Unit, Eindhoven. Seated l. to r. Sister Vaughan-Jones, Major Fitzgibbon, Sister i/c theatre, Major Hodgson, the author. Standing l. to r. Major Holland, 2nd Anaesthetist, Major Irwin, Captain Gibson

and the sooner it was off the better. The surgery was the quickest and the most efficient that I had ever known and in no time at all we had the soldier in the ward under our care.

We did not notice the lengthening of the day. It was so dark anyway in the tent that we needed electric light for most of the time, but now Audrey and Barbara were there, fresh from sleep, ready to take over. Joan and I were all at once aware that we were desperately tired. We explained what had been done and what remained to be done, and reached for tin hats and ground-sheets. There was a hot meal waiting for us in the Mess, then the ambulance would take us to the convent at La Deliverande. The rain had stopped but everything dripped. Apple trees showered us unkindly as we made our way to the dining tent. The ground shook and rumbled beneath our feet and the sky flashed angrily to the great guns that were going off not so very far away. We were the lucky ones, however. Major Edwards and his team operated all through the night.

The road to La Deliverande was breaking up under random shelling and our progress was slow and bumpy. The barrage on our right, the driver told us, was directed at the air strip. On our left, exploding shells lit up the sky over Caen.

Caen must be taken. The Allied line in this sector could not advance until a way past this hub of enemy resistance was found. The offensive launched that morning was part of a move to encircle the town but before the 49th Division could establish bridgeheads over the two rivers, Odon and Orne, the heavily fortified heights of Rauray Ridge would have to be cleared and the battles would be fierce and bloody.

It was nearly ten o'clock when we rattled over the cobbles of the deserted main street of La Deliverande. The folk here had seen bitter fighting in the early days of the campaign and, now that the Allied armies had passed by, they were content to go thankfully to bed with the sun. Our driver put us down by a pair of stout wooden doors set in a wall beneath a great bell.

'You have to give that a pull,' he said. 'See you 0700 hrs.' He put the ambulance into a 'U' turn and headed back to Herman-ville. The silence of the village closed around us. We looked at the bell hanging there above us, took a deep breath and pulled on the rope. The clamour was appalling. Surely someone must have heard? I yawned loudly for I was nearly asleep on my feet, and at the same time a wooden shutter clapped back from a grille set in the door, making both of us start.

'Qui va là?' It was a deep Brünnhilde of a voice.

'Deux infermières Anglaises,' we squeaked.

The door was opened. A middle-aged woman dressed in the habit of a religious order stood holding a lantern. She ushered us in while she locked the door and slid the wooden bar into position. Dimly, we could distinguish the shadowy arches of a cloister and a tormented Christ hanging from a cross. Kilduff or Annie P. Scott would have been more at home here.

'Venez,' she swished ahead of us, her bunch of keys muted in the deep folds of her garment, and led us, thudding heavily after her in our gumboots, to an inner courtyard where she drew our attention to a cast-iron pump and bucket. In the further-most corner of the courtyard, a single light flickered in a small, high-ceilinged room. This was where we were to sleep.

'Dormez-bien, mes enfants.' She turned away, lifting her lamp for a moment to indicate a vague direction. 'La toilette au fond du jardin,' and she bobbed away into the dark.

I shivered and bent to light the 'Beatrice' made ready for us by Audrey and Barbara. They had also made up our beds and left half a tin of milk with some coffee beside our mess-tins.

'Now all we have to do,' said Joan, 'is to brave the pump and find la toilette.'

The ornate bower in the garden was approached by a flight of steps, and it was more like an altar than a lavatory. We were overcome by a fit of the giggles. Ablutions at the pump were hilarious. We lost half the soap down the drain and I was terri-fied in case my one false tooth followed it. The water was ice-cold, and black and silver by moonlight, but we were able to wash away the clinging smells of the ward and felt warm and relaxed afterwards as we sat drinking coffee.

'I wish we'd been able to finish all the dressings.' We spoke in whispers, as if the saints in their niches in the wall might eavesdrop. The clink of a teaspoon chimed like a bell in that holy room.

'There's tomorrow.'

'And the next day. Bloody war.'

To be able to talk like this with a friend made it all bearable. If we had stopped to think too deeply, we would have been drained by the tragedy of it all. We were young, and youth is very sensible of how much pathos it can take. Older women, I think, would not have survived without scars. We had a last cigarette and crept into our bedrolls. Above us, St. Francis and his birds trembled all night long with the distant gunfire, shaking down a snow of plaster that covered us as we slept.

It seemed that we had just dropped off to sleep when we were awakened by the persistent tolling of a bell from deep within the convent. Reluctantly, we shuffled out of our bedrolls and prepared to dress. Another clean shirt. There had to be a washing day soon. The A.V.s lasted forever.

The only acceptable undress for ablutions at the pump was rolled-up sleeves with collar undone, for we were now surrounded by modest young novices, with their long, full skirts pinned back, sweeping up the courtyard. Wary of our trousers, they returned our smiles shyly and looked the other way while we sluiced in the tingling water. A lark soared high above us in a bright and windy sky. Yesterday's rain had gone and, with it, our despondency.

There was a pot of coffee, bread and apricot jam waiting for us in our austere little cell when we returned from washing and we sat in the early sunshine, eating breakfast to the sound of unaccompanied voices drifting over the courtyard in a hymn to the glory of God. The world seemed full of promise.

We passed through the door into the street just as the first customers of the day were leaving the boulangerie with loaves of black bread under their arms. An old woman with a child by her side prodded a fat cow to milking and washing danced at the back of the houses. La Deliverande was up and doing and Joan and I drew many curious glances as we stood at the side of the road waiting for our transport. Again, it was the trousers that baffled the passers-by; the inhabitants of La Deliverande did not know whether to laugh at us or cry for us.

The F.D.S., when we reached it, was drying out. Everything was happening in the orchard behind the church. The men from Searchlights were hopefully washing their socks, and wet blankets flapped from branches of the trees. Pioneers were laying fresh rubble in the worst of the muddy ruts and the damp canvas of the ward tent bellied in the fresh breeze. Inside smelt sweet and clean. Yesterday's foulness was blown away and Duncan gave us a cheery 'Good morning' as he swept the tarpaulin floor. It seemed to us that the men on their stretchers looked a little less grey, a little more alert. There was colour in some faces, and the beginnings of interest in their surroundings and in us. As we stood by the entrance listening to the night report from Audrey and Barbara, we watched the man with the fractured pelvis who barely opened his eyes yesterday. He was fumbling for the little cotton drawstring bag known as a 'Dorothy Bag' which was tied to the handle of each man's stretcher and held his paybook and personal possessions. Now he took out a comb and painstakingly began to put in order that part of his hair within his reach. We felt greatly encouraged.

It had been a noisy night, the night shift told us. The gun in the nearby field had blasted away without ceasing. More casualties had been admitted but even with more wounded to look after, the new day went well for us. We slipped into an unhurried routine, confident that most of the men were responding to treatment. One man with a severe abdominal wound had died in the night but most of the others stood a fair chance of recovery. On his round of the patients, Major Edwards expressed his satisfaction and several of the transfusions were discontinued.

As the men improved, the question of diet began to concern us. In a field cookhouse such as ours, there was only the sketchiest of cooking potential. Our menu was restricted to tinned foods. Tins of stew, beans, bacon, sausages and various fruits were not the best invalid diet. There was no bread yet for army bakers had not at that time crossed the Channel and the ships' biscuits on which we continued to break our teeth were quite out of the question for sick men. Yet, as the intravenous fluids were discontinued, nourishing food was of the utmost importance.

The best we could do was to strain the gravy from tins of stew and thicken this with a little potato. We followed this with minced tinned fruit. There was plenty of tinned milk so we were able to make nourishing drinks such as Horlicks, Ovaltine and cocoa. We longed for eggs. With eggs at our disposal, we could make all manner of easily digested meals on the small primus stove in the ward tent.

Lunchtime was a lengthy business as we fed those able to take solid food, slow teaspoonful by teaspoonful. We were engaged on this one day when we had a visit from the area padre. He was a bright-eyed little man with rosy cheeks who drove a very battered old jeep at great speed around his 'parish'.

'Come to see if I can offer you any medical comforts,' he said as he slithered down the ward entrance. 'Hot water bottles. Pneumonia jackets.'

We had no use for either of these items but we told him of our concern about diets and our need for eggs. The problem intrigued him. Here was an occasion when his knowledge of the locality could be put to real use. The nearby farms, he suggested, must surely have a surplus of eggs now that the German messes had retreated. From his own observation, he knew that in many of the farms there were civilians who had been injured in the bombing, though not seriously enough to merit a bed in the French hospital at Bayeux. Why should we not treat these minor casualties in return for eggs?

'As out-patients, of course,' he said.

Our first reaction was to dismiss the suggestion out of hand. We had enough to do without taking on out-patients, but then we stopped to consider. 'Perhaps a few?'

'Say, half an hour every morning?'

'No need for two of us. One could carry on with the hard work.'

The vision of eggs was tempting and we made up our minds

to give the scheme a try. Since the Major would be obliged to refuse permission if we asked him, we decided to go ahead, and call it all off if he objected.

No more than six, we told the padre, to come at eleven-thirty next morning on the understanding that, if casualties arrived, the deal was off. Delighted to be of help, he took off in his jeep, promising eggs for tomorrow.

'Sister! Resus. is full of Frenchies!' said Duncan excitedly the next morning, signalling urgently from the end of the ward. 'They've brought eggs but they won't part with them.'

Joan was down on her knees on the tarpaulin dressing a wound of buttock. She nodded towards me. 'You go. Your French is better than mine.'

I set a tray with instruments and dressings and begged a small steriliser from the theatre. 'Out-patients,' I explained to Duncan, 'in return for eggs.'

They stood, apprehensive and ill at ease, amongst the drip stands and oxygen cylinders of the resuscitation annexe, holding their egg offerings close. There was an old man with a grubby bandage over one eye, another with his arm in a sling, and two women with a young boy clinging to their skirts, a child with enormous eyes who promptly began to howl at the sight of me, swathed in a towel, my face half-hidden by a mask. I seated them on blood boxes and lit the spirit lamp under the steriliser, wondering what I would find beneath those dirty bits of bandage.

The boy had a glancing shrapnel wound just below the knee and the soiled rag stuck fast. In anticipation of the worst, he began to howl again and his mother clutched him to her defensively, so I gave him a bowl of antiseptic lotion and a swab of cotton wool and showed him how to soak off the dressing himself. He was soon concentrating so hard on not hurting himself that he forgot to cry. His grandmother had burnt her arm at the kitchen stove. She had spent most of her life hand-in-hand with disaster and her face showed it. She lived now with her daughter-in-law, guarding the little boy, Marc, who was the last surviving male in the family.

One of the old men had brick dust in his eye and the other a fractured collarbone. The whole party took no more than half an hour and, for this, my grateful patients, reassured now and quite at ease, were pleased to fill my tin hat with eggs. The thought occurred to me that they might be interested to see the ward. Perhaps these peasants who had suffered from the Allied invasion should see our soldiers who were so grievously wounded in the fight for freedom?

I beckoned them to follow me around the side of the tent, over the guy ropes to the ward entrance, surprising a Pioneer busy there with spade and shovel. Hastily he stood aside to let us pass and stared in disbelief as the procession of black shawls, berets and sabots followed me into the ward.

Duncan, who was going from bed to bed with cups of Bovril, patently did not approve of these goings on. 'Mornin' all,' he said heavily, just loud enough to make a protest. What next, he was no doubt thinking, and what'll the Major say?

The visitors looked at Joan, busy with penicillin and syringe, and at the men on stretchers. 'Ah, les pauvres blessés . . .' The war-weary grandmother rocked herself to and fro in remembered anguish and the old men clicked their teeth. Then, quietly, all withdrew.

There was never any shortage of eggs after that. They brought other delicacies too, good, wholesome broth and jellied consommè and savoury custards. A few days later, when Major Edwards chanced upon the little out-patients clinic, he noted the array of offerings and discreetly retired, deciding that this was something he had better not know about.

Evacuations from the F.D.S. were still impossible. Shelling of the landing strips continued and the road back to La Deliverande was collecting more than its usual share of sporadic shells. It was soon decided that it would be safer, on the whole, for us to stay at the F.D.S. and our sleeping arrangements at the convent came to an end.

'Then you'll have to be dug in,' said the Major, who was refreshingly avuncular towards us. 'In the orchard. A long way from any rude soldiery.'

A couple of Pioneers were set to digging out a rectangular area, half of which was more deeply excavated than the other. This section, which was about three feet deep and roofed over with rough planks, housed snugly two camp beds alongside each other. The remaining space at the higher level accommodated our tin trunks and stoves. A tent was erected overall. A few yards away among the apple trees was what looked like a hessian telephone box and a freshly dug heap of earth. We fixed up a washing line and invited the M.O.s for a house-warming with our N.A.A.F.I. ration of gin. At the Major's instigation a painted sign appeared at the approaches to our new home. 'Sisters' Quarters. Keep Out.' This was quickly followed by a similar sign near the Engineers' tents. 'Brothers' Quarters. Come In.'

With no time wasted in travelling, our day at the F.D.S. became easier and the four of us had no difficulty in managing the work. Only a trickle of casualties was coming through as most of the action was going on west of Caen. Even so, the ward tent was crammed. Of the men who had been there since our arrival, most were making good progress and wounds were healing. They were giving us a little light-hearted back-chat now, which was always a good sign, but there were those who did not recover and a few more white wooden crosses appeared in the corner of the field behind the tents. The padre hated this part of his job. There were times when his cheerful spirit deserted him. He was much more deeply concerned about casualties than one would have supposed from his light-hearted manner and sometimes we would surprise him, standing at the foot of a stretcher, a look of misery on his face, confronted with his inability to help a man injured in the firing line, where he would never be.

Every night was firework night at the F.D.S. The sky above our orchard dug-out was spanned with leaping tracers but although the guns in the next field banged away without cease, they did not prevent Joan and me from sleeping soundly in the two beds still warm from Audrey and Barbara. In the morning we would discover small beetles and fragments of earth lodged in the cold cream on our faces, shaken down from our bedroom ceiling by the reverberations of the guns. We did not see much of the other shift since, if we were not on duty, we were usually asleep, although sometimes after supper in the Mess, Joan and I would have a game of darts with the men before turning in for the night. Bath night, we were to learn later, was greatly appreciated. Then, our perfectly thrown silhouettes, each with a foot in a biscuit tin and wearing nothing at all but a tin hat, were revealed on the side of the tent by the glare of our Tilly lamp.

At last there was a sea evacuation. The German battery which had been causing all the trouble was put out of action and we could start moving patients. When it came to preparing men for evacuation, Duncan was on home ground. Methodically and efficiently, he wrapped up the lucky ones who were going home, tied their medical notes to their pyjamas and checked that paybooks were in their Dorothy Bags. Joan and I dressed their wounds for the last time.

'Goodbye, Sis. Thanks for everything.' They were chirpy now, hardly able to believe they were going home, a destination that had seemed doubtful at times. The fact that some would have to face further operations, or that some had a limb less than when they started, did not seem to dim their excitement at going. We were as happy as they were, remembering their condition on our arrival.

The F.D.S. could function properly now with evacuations proceeding smoothly and there was no longer any need for nursing sisters. There was an additional reason for wanting us out of the area, for a full-scale, head-on attack on Caen was imminent. It seemed the only way to overcome this persistently resistant obstacle. A major offensive was planned for 8th July to be preceded the night before by an air attack of such ferocity that the defences of Caen would be wiped out, thus leaving the way clear for our armour to go in and take the town once and for all.

Our own hospital, the 75th B.G.H., was given a site with instructions to become operational immediately and all sisters were recalled to base. On the morning of the 7th July we said goodbye to our friends at the Field Dressing Station and to our home in the earth in the orchard.

8

'Harley Street'

Our new hospital site was on the Bayeux-Caen road on a stretch that later came to be known as 'Harley Street' when many more hospitals joined us there, but on the morning of the 7th July it looked as though the circus had come to town. Packing cases were strewn about like a child's bricks in the large field not far from Bayeux and marquees reared up shakily on their guy ropes. The men of our unit, stripped to the waist, hammered in tent pegs and assembled the ridge poles of what were to be the wards. Smithy, the Company Officer, strode about with a whistle in his mouth followed by Pioneers carrying buckets of white-wash to mark the edges of the roads that were being laid as fast as trucks could deliver the rubble to make them with. Rows of latrines were taking up position behind a hessian screen in the long grass. Field incinerators belched black smoke from their diet of cardboard and straw. Signposts pointed the way to the cookhouse, which was already producing tea and baked beans, to the Hospital Office, a confusion of trestle tables and papers, and to the Mortuary, as yet a bundle of sacking by the edge of the wood.

The Matron, Miss Ellen Davies, anxiously ticked off the names of her nursing staff as we returned from our various post-ings and set about unpacking equipment. This was the day she had been waiting for. Since landing two weeks ago on 22nd June, she had been assisting in the administration of the 81st B.G.H. while waiting for a site for her own hospital. Other hospitals had come out from England in the meantime. The 88th, 77th, 79th and the 20th B.G.H. had all been able to claim their planned positions but our allocated placement on the Caen plain was still in enemy hands. Now, we had a tight schedule. There was no light yet, no sewerage and the roads were not finished but we must be prepared for casualties the next day, 8th July.

With claw hammers, scissors and knives, we attacked the crates we had packed in Watford. Spurred by the urgency of the situation, clerks helped to put up beds. The Quartermaster doled out pillows, sheets and blankets, towels and pyjamas. Everybody lent a hand where it was most needed. The surgical instruments which we had so efficiently greased against rust had to be cleaned and boiled as soon as the sterilisers could be located. Hypodermic syringes, number one priority, must be ready for instant use and, since this was before the day of the disposable, plastic syringe, glass body and steel plunger had to be wrapped in gauze and gently brought to the boil before use. All these procedures took time but the job at Watford had been well done and unpacking went smoothly. Everything was where it should be, though one parcel marked 'Sphygmomanometer' contained two Union Jacks and a bicycle pump.

In the event, our first casualties came sooner than expected. The ground attack on Caen was not due to take place till the following morning but Canadian troops, making a preliminary probe to test the defences of the perimeter of the town, met with unexpectedly strong resistance and were our first patients.

Joan and I, together again in Resus., were still searching for the morphia when the first stretchers were carried through the doorway of our brand-new tent. In the wards, the last pillows were being pushed into covers and lines were being drawn up in Admission Books. Miraculously, the Engineers got the dynamo going right on time and the hospital sprang into light. Miss Davies did a quick round of the wards. The 75th was ready for action.

The light had almost faded from the sky when a huge spread of Halifaxes and Lancasters flew overhead, bound for Caen to drop several thousand tons of explosive. The burning town coloured the sky an angry red and the ground beneath our feet trembled as load after load of bombs rained down on Caen. The ground attack began the next day but the very success of the previous night's bombardment now hindered our troops. The roads through the town were choked with mountains of rubble that no armour could penetrate. German troops, driven from the centre, now took up positions in the sturdy stone houses on the outskirts, converting each one into a blockhouse, so the way past Caen was still closed to us.

From the moment that the attack began, we, in the 75th, were inundated with casualties whose evacuation had to be organised with the same speed as their reception. The busiest recorded day was the 18th July when 446 wounded were admitted, and on the same day 328 post-operative cases were evacuated to the United Kingdom. There was barely time for us to sit down for a meal. It was work–sleep, work–sleep. In Resus. we admitted one convoy after another. There was no need for Joan and me to speak. We worked as a team in a tent that was never empty.

Again and again they came, through the day and night, men with different faces, different names but the same terrible injuries: the lieutenant needing urgent amputation of both shattered legs, the tank commander baked like a potato in his burning tank, the sergeant with the piece of mortar lodged in his carotid artery. It was a high price in casualties for a few miles of advance.

The wounded were not all British. Wounded German P.O.W.s were beginning to filter through on their way to the marshalling 'cages' before being shipped to Britain. Some of these men were from the S.S. Hitler's élite fighting corps. I cannot forget my first encounter with a stormtrooper.

The greater part of a newly arrived convoy of wounded had come to us in Resus. and the tent was packed. Joan was accompanying Lt. Colonel Harding as he made out his theatre list while I entered new arrivals in the Admission Book. As I stepped over the stretchers laid out on the tarpaulin, my attention was drawn to one field-grey uniform amongst all the khaki. The British soldiers all around him were too seriously injured to notice their odd companion and too desperate to care. He was a tall young man. His one remaining leg overhung the stretcher by several inches. A bloodied dressing covered the stump of the other leg. With eyes tight closed and a face taut with pain, he whispered 'Wasser, wasser,' as I passed.

The fact that he was an enemy did not really register with me. A nurse's training of caring cannot be switched on and off like a light so I fetched some water and went down on my knees to slide a hand under his damp, blonde hair and hold the feeding cup to his lips. On the collar of his jacket was the forked-lightning flash of the SS.

He drank thirstily and opened light blue eyes. They were blank until he focused on my battledress. Then I saw his expression change. With a convulsive jerk, he spat fair and square in my face.

'English pig!'

My stomach turned over and I thought I would be sick. I let his sweaty head fall back and went to plunge my fouled-up face in a basin of cold water.

'Bloody Kraut,' grumbled the orderly.

'Leave that man till last,' called out Colonel Harding in a voice hard with anger. 'There are more urgent cases.'

Although I scrubbed my face with a nailbrush until it smarted I could not remove the feel of that German's hate. Other German casualties came later, not fanatics like this one, but ordinary men grateful for medical attention. They tempered that first brutal impression of a German soldier.

During this early part of July, the Normandy bridgehead was consolidating only very slowly. Advances were in bitterly con-tested yards with high casualties. On our right, the Americans, in a push south-west to reach the sea across the neck of the Cotentin peninsula, were struggling with swamps and flooded river valleys and, further east, their efforts to take the enemy strongpoint at St. Lô were meeting with no success as yet. In the British sector, the head-on trial of strength went on against the deep German defences on the outskirts of Caen. Convoys of ambulances making for the hospitals were unending. We sisters saw each other briefly at mealtimes or before bed.

I have memories of a huge appetite. Rations were plentiful and filling, if not exactly Cordon Bleu, and they received a great fillip one day when a dusty young man on a motorbike, bear-ing a sack of loaves on his back, appeared outside the Sisters' mess asking for me. It was Ray Dobson, ex-medical student from the Royal Victoria Infirmary, now a lieutenant in the R.A.M.C. He had been to Arromanches with casualties and had come upon our old friend, Russell Slater who was M.O. on board the vessel that was taking the wounded men.

'He sent this load of bread for you. "Find the 75th," he says. "The poor girl's probably starving."'

We were suitably grateful. After weeks of ships' biscuits, ordinary bread tasted like the purest confection. We took Ray into the Mess, fed him and made a fuss of him before sending him on his way to his First Aid Post further up the line.

Russell sent news of the Newcastle hospital. He had paid a visit there on his last leave and found V.A.D. nurses (Voluntary Aid Detachment of the Red Cross) helping on all the wards so, for once, there was plenty of staff. Perhaps the war had done some good, for it would be difficult to go back to the bad old days when a staff of four nurses had to look after sometimes as many as forty patients.

There were geordies from 50 Div. in the wards, men who had landed on 'Gold' beach on D-Day, men wounded at the battles for Le Hamel and Tilly-sur-Seulles, some of whom must have passed through our hands at the 75th. They had survived the chain of medical units and the subsequent Channel crossing to come home at last.

Russell's bread was particularly welcomed by Sister Darby who ran our Mess and did her best to make us comfortable. She was somewhat older than the rest of us and when I look back to the difficult conditions we lived under at that time I am filled with admiration for the older nurses who were amongst us. Most of us were young and could fall asleep on a clothes-line, but I wonder how I would have coped if I had been forty-five instead of twenty-five, with perhaps a touch of rheumatism or a fickle bladder? I blush to think that we never considered their possible discomfort. There was no privacy whatever in the latrines which were simply one continuous line of wooden seaters. The Matron, coming in behind the hessian screen one day, misinterpreted Annie P.'s getting to her feet as a gesture of respect, when she was, in fact, about to leave.

'That's all right, Sister,' the Matron said in all seriousness. 'No need for that in here.'

'When is a Matron not a Matron?' Annie regaled us with the story. 'When she's next to you on the john.'

I was sharing a tent with a Welsh Sister at this time, black-haired Kay Minor. Her sing-song and my Geordie accent kept sympathetic company. Duff joined us one night as we brewed our usual nightcap before turning in. She was looking all bottled up.

'There's this Canadian,' she began. We pushed the tin of N.A.A.F.I. cigarettes nearer and handed her a coffee. 'I find him crying, stuffing the sheet into his mouth so that no-one will hear. I heard his bed shaking.' Kay and I sat quiet. 'He'd just escaped from the Germans. His fingers are in an awful mess. They'd driven sharp bits of wood under his nails to make him talk.' One's whole mind cringed.

Two weeks later, on a fine, warm night when most of us were sleeping with the tent flaps open in our corner of the field, well away from the rest of the unit, I awoke to the sound of voices, and made out the vague shape of a man in uniform crouched outside the tent by the head of Kay's bed. In my drowsy state, I imagined it to be some boy friend of Kay's but the sheer improbability of any boy friend, be he ever so eager, daring to set foot in our Holy of Holies, roused me to a clear head. Kay was speaking, quite calmly, in a low, insistent whisper. 'Go away. You mustn't come in here.'

I sat up, now wide-awake. 'What's going on?'

Still in a hoarse whisper, for it was around one o'clock in the morning, Kay explained. 'He's as drunk as a fiddler's bitch and he won't go away.'

'Who is he?'

'How the hell do I know!'

I decided to take a hand. 'Get out of here,' I said, very firmly. 'Go back where you came from.'

My intervention had the opposite to the desired effect for the man decided to investigate the interior of the tent, coming in on all fours like a blundering animal. He made straight for my bed and wrenched off the blankets. My instinctive response surprised even myself. It must have been some memory of those self-defence lessons way back in Scotland, for I swung my clenched fist straight into his face. I don't flatter myself that there was any weight behind the punch but he was, as Kay had said, very drunk indeed, and he toppled over on to his back. In a flash, Kay and I were on him, pinning down his arms.

'Bull's-eye, Mac,' she breathed admiringly.

There was no need to raise the alarm. We had made a fair bit of noise with our scuffling and he had been in other tents before ours. An odd little company was already hurrying over the field towards our tent; the Matron, caught in her curlers, the Colonel with his greatcoat over his pyjamas and a Staff Sergeant holding high a hurricane lantern. The intruder, it appeared, with proper respect for rank had called upon the Matron first of all!

He had never looked like becoming dangerous and the poor befuddled fellow was led away and put under guard. In the morning, we learnt the sad story. It was Duff's Canadian who had been sent to convalesce at the Rest Centre in Bayeux after leaving our hospital. Before returning to his unit at the front, he wanted to say thank you to the sister who had been so kind to him. A shot of Calvados, the fiery local liqueur, had given him Dutch courage, but he had made the mistake of continuing halfway down the bottle, and arrived at our camp very much the worse for wear, when all the day staff were asleep. Kay and I had brought to a halt his systematic search through the tents for Duff. She went to see him in the Guard tent, and when the story was explained to the C.O., our intruder got off with a caution and a bottle of aspirin.

Deeply involved as we all were with the wounded men in our care, no-one noticed that one of the medical staff was under strain. At first light, one misty morning, a stretcher bearing a body draped in a Union Jack was carried from the medical officers' tents. Major MacPherson had shared a tent with Capt.

Lloyd and had been awakened by the shot. He was shaken now and bitterly self-critical. How was it possible to share a tent with a man and not know he had this on his mind?

But we had all been too busy with our own jobs to stand back and look about us. No-one had realised that Capt. Lloyd, a true physician, had been overwhelmed by a sense of failure amongst the need for so much surgery. Nobody here had pneumonia or nephritis, or, if they had, it was secondary to all the surgery. His day would have come again if he had waited. In a little while, plenty of men would have been grateful for his care.

The aerial bombing and head-on attack on Caen had been only partially successful. Our wards full of casualties were the cost of clearing no more than the centre and the north of the town. All the land to the east of the town and the southern suburbs were still in German hands. On 18th July, a new offensive was launched by our armoured divisions, successfully cutting a swathe east and south of Caen, through some of Hitler's most experienced troops, the 21st Panzers, 1st and 12th S.S. Panzers. At the same time, the Canadians attacked the garrisoned suburbs and systematically cleared them of their stubborn defenders. The whole of Caen was in our hands at last.

Throughout these weeks in July, our stretchers in Resus. were never empty for long, but only a few of the faces remain with me. Most of the men brought there were too badly wounded to communicate. Individual characteristics became blurred in men wounded so critically. I remember the continuous challenge of falling blood pressures, and the terrible haemorrhages when blood dripped to the tarpaulin floor at a faster rate than we could pour it into a vein. I remember the tell-tale bubbly feeling of flesh that told of the presence of gasgangrene, but I remember too the miracle of a grey face turning pink. Strangely, and mercifully, I have forgotten the deaths, though one bright face I do remember. He was brought into our tent with eyes wide open, looking about him, still remembering to be polite.

'I've often wondered what you sisters got up to,' he said, with a brave, cheeky smile. Then a sudden look of surprise opened his

eyes very wide and he was dead, still with the smile on his lips.
A captain of the Coldstream Guards, the same age as myself, he
was caught unawares by death. With part of a shell buried in his
back, he had suddenly tweaked his spinal cord and, in one
astonished moment, he was gone.

I realised that I needed a break from Resus. when I lost my
self-control over a tin of peaches. Tinned fruit was in short
supply and could be had only on a requisition form from the
Q.M. for those genuinely sick men who could not eat suet
pudding and prunes. One day, when an unknown M.O. who
was temporarily attached to our unit helped himself to a tin of
peaches from our precious store in Resus., I suddenly saw red.
To my very aggressive demands that he should return the tin
immediately, he laughed lightheartedly and made off with his
loot. I rushed off to speak to the Matron.

'He's stolen a tin of peaches from my patients,' I proclaimed
and instantly started to cry, with tears of rage against the
wicked M.O. and tears of chagrin that I should cry. Very
wisely, the Matron moved me to another department, a ward
recently taken over by a visiting head-injuries team under the
C.O., Major 'Sam' Small.

After the constant activity of Resus., 'Heads' was as tranquil
as a cathedral. Its occupants were brought here straight from
the special head-injuries theatre, each wearing a protective
plaster-of-Paris helmet, and they lay for days in deep, post-
operative coma before finally surfacing to recovery.

It was the beginning of August now and the weather turned
hot. Our hardest job in 'Heads' was keeping men cool whose
heat-regulating machinery in the brain had been impaired. I
was working with Janet Smart here, and we were continually
sponging their inert bodies in order to keep down soaring temperatures. The sides of the tent were rolled up to catch any cross
breezes and we ourselves had put away A.V.s and were once
more in grey cotton frocks. Because of the heat, our patients lay
naked under a loose sheet and frequently caused us embarrassment, one way and another, as on the occasion when one of the
men, deeply comatosed until now, suddenly, quietly, nipped out

of bed, and, before we could shout for an orderly, was away under the tent side, stark naked except for his plaster helmet. He was retrieved within minutes and led back to bed, quite unrepentant.

'Ah, Sister,' he greeted Janet, red-faced and shushing. 'Have you ever been to India?'

'How can you shame me like that, Captain Robertson,' she demanded as we tucked him into bed again and gave him a sedative. 'In front of the whole hospital!' But Capt. Robertson was literally out of his mind at the time and when he eventually recovered, would never have believed the story.

'They're gay rude sometimes,' Janet confided to me with twitching lips.

There was the burly Guards Major who had been sniped. He was brought from the theatre in a very boisterous mood and it took the surgeon, an orderly, Janet and me to get him into bed and keep him there. Then he started singing. In a deep and penetrating voice he sang clearly and distinctly all the words of a song whose melody was familiar but whose lyrics most certainly were not, and would have been more at home in a rugby football changing room. Sam Small, the surgeon, was about to make a hasty retreat when an amazing transformation took place in the ward. One by one, the unconscious men, responding to the barrack room choruses, joined in till the whole tent resounded. Still with eyes closed and lying totally immobile like rows of white-capped angels, our ward full of head injuries rollicked through every verse.

Hopping about in embarrassment, we tried to quieten them, and ticked off the orderly for laughing, but we could do nothing about the broad grin on Sam Small's face.

'You two girls really must not excite these poor men so,' he said and went back to the theatre in guffaws.

'Heads' differed from Resus. in that there were no open wounds for us to deal with, no dramatic shock treatment, but the nursing care was very intensive. Each man was fed by nasal tube with egg and milk, casein or glucose. A detailed chart of fluid intake and output was kept so that there could be no possibility of dehydration. This was a very real danger when the men sweated so much in hot weather. We had to change their positions regularly to prevent sores forming on their vulnerable, flaccid flesh and check that they were never left on a wet sheet. The mouth was an ever-present source of infection without the natural cleansing function of eating and the production of salivary juices. Coagulations and crusts had to be continually removed from the gums of men who lay snoring with open mouths for most of the time. Flies made our job that much harder. To keep them off, we made little masks of gauze to lay over the men's defenceless faces. The reward was to see consciousness returning, to be able to remove a nasal tube and spoon minced chicken into a suddenly hungry mouth beneath wide-awake eyes. After that came the glad evacuation to the United Kingdom.

The warm weather that was so trying for the head injuries was also plaguing our infantry as they slogged through the dust on the road to Falaise, south of Caen. While British thrusts in this direction continued to engage the main part of Hitler's armour, the Americans opened a major offensive in the west. St. Lô was taken at last and they were able to advance in a great leap across Brittany to the coast. Soon the Allied armies would join up and wheel eastward, using Caen as a pivot, making for the Seine gap and Paris. Now, at last, we were breaking out of the tight little bridgehead.

More hospitals were arriving from England to take their share of casualties and we at the 75th began to feel our workload eased. There were off-duty periods for us now and we were able to lie in the sun in the privacy of our enclosure by the wood and do nothing. Nearby army messes were very indulgent with us, arranging a party whenever three or four Q.A.s could be gathered together. There were not a lot of women around and our company was much sought after. Inevitably, whirlwind romances developed before the men moved up the line.

One of the sisters caught up in this way was Mary MacDonald from the Highlands, a good-looking, stately girl with thick, black hair and full red lips. A calm, reposeful girl who listened more than she talked, she was not the kind to be swept off her feet but before a certain Artillery captain moved away, he asked her to become engaged and she agreed. As the kind of girl who did not easily give away her heart, she was utterly devastated by the news a little while later that he had been killed in action. A dispatch rider brought his personal effects to her, all that she had to remember him by. But it was even harder for her the following day when an agitated padre appeared in a dusty jeep asking for Sister MacDonald. Someone had made a mistake in sending the deceased captain's effects to Mary. They should have gone to his next-of-kin, namely, his wife.

Mary removed her own letters from the bundle of the captain's things and gave it back to the padre. The captain was later discovered to have engaged himself to a young French woman in addition to Mary. It had been a bad habit of his.

9

Bayeux: The Break-out

Bayeux was a Rest Centre for troops of the line. Men in uniform crowded its narrow pavements, American blacks from the Deep South rubbing shoulders with Irish Guards, Canadians and Poles; its little shops tempted us with perfume, silk stockings, apple tarts and trashy jewellery. The troops' spell away from the fighting was brief so there was always a good deal of merry-making in Bayeux, with cider, cognac and Calvados. Our radiologist, Lt. Peter Tait, got wind of a convent there where one could take a bath for a very small fee. We were more than a little interested since none of us had washed in anything bigger than a biscuit tin for about seven weeks now, and when Peter turned up with borrowed transport for the expedition, those of us who were off duty, which included Pin, Duff and me, eagerly joined him, equipped with soap and towel.

We were not the only ones to hear about the nuns' public-spirited gesture. In the drive leading to the convent we found parked vehicles of all descriptions with every imaginable divisional sign. Servicemen of all ranks and units sat in the long grass near a semi-circle of steaming, whitewashed cells. We took our place amongst brigadiers and corporals, commandos and caterers, pioneers and padres, each carrying a rolled-up towel and a piece of soap.

As soon as a bath hut was vacated, a lay sister appeared with a cloth and basin to prepare it for the next occupant who was already breathing down her neck, and as we settled ourselves to wait our turn we prayed that the hot water would not run out.

'Great occasion,' said the colonel who moved up to make room for Pin and me.

'Better than a biscuit tin,' Pin agreed.

He looked at her in some surprise. 'Lucky you to have a biscuit tin.'

I glanced at Pin and saw her nose twitch.

When it was my turn, I paid my francs to the sister and closed the door of the hut behind me. A deep and narrow copper bath, burnished like red gold, stood stark against whitewashed walls. There was a duckboard and a chair and that was all. I tore off my clothes, rashly tipped in the whole of my Worth's bath essence and stepped reverently into the steam. None but those who have gone without hot water for seven weeks will understand the sheer, voluptuous luxury of that first Bayeux bath.

I wanted to lie there and soak for hours, but after too short a time, I reluctantly pulled out the plug. Duff, too, was evidently finding the water irresistible and, as I went back to the others, I heard her launch into a full-throated rendering of 'One Fine Day'. She had a nice voice and the bath hut made an ideal echo chamber but her audience was growing restive. A nuggetty Geordie from 50 Div., sitting on his hunkers and smoking a tab end, was all for cutting it short.

'Get yersell weshed, hinny,' he advised in a penetrating corncrake of a voice. 'Divvent worry aboot the consort.'

On the way back through Bayeux, we stopped at Le Lion d'Or for a cup of ersatz coffee. It was ground from acorns and tasted like stewed boots, but it was fun to sit at the rusty iron tables with their chipped marble tops and watch the Press boys come and go. This hotel was their H.Q. and there was usually a bit of drama going on. Today was no exception. Men wearing the green flash of the Press hurried by with copy in their hands. Agitated small groups conferred in low voices.

'Something big is on.' Peter Tait looked knowledgeable. 'We'll catch it tomorrow.'

The next day brought as many German wounded as British. The American front had now swung round and was advancing eastwards towards Le Mans. British troops driving south to Falaise completed the perfect pincer movement and a whole German army was caught in the Falaise pocket.

The Germans who now streamed through our hospitals were not the proud *herrenvolk* of earlier days but middle-aged men with ulcers and boys of sixteen. Hitler was beginning to feel a manpower shortage and had just reduced the call-up age.

The 'Heads' unit left our hospital now to move further up the line and I joined Soutie on one of the surgical wards which had its share of wounded Germans. We found it difficult to look upon these sixteen-year-olds as enemies; schoolboys, they were, not soldiers. As I dressed their wounds, I reflected how their mothers must be worrying about them, wounded and about to be sent to some place of captivity in hostile England.

Our 'office' was the bridging annexe between a tent full of P.O.W.s and a regular British ward, and as we went from one to the other, we could not fail to notice, with some amusement, the vastly differing characteristics of each ward. There was a relaxed, easy relationship with our own men, for the Tommy, if he was not actually breathing his last, was perky and cheeky but never disrespectful and we needed no rules of conduct. The Germans, however, expected rules, looked for instruction as to what might or might not be done, and were nonplussed when they found none.

The first convoy of prisoners had been admitted no more than an hour before the Germans had appointed a tent-'meister' amongst themselves. It was his duty to screech '*Achtung!*' every time a sister or the M.O. appeared on the ward, with the astonishing result that everyone who had two good feet clapped them together to attention as he lay in bed.

Soutie soon put a stop to this, with a firm 'Mother-knows-best' smile on her face. 'We'll have none of your nasty Nazi habits here,' she said, to the prisoner in the first bed. 'Turn over.' And she rammed home 3000 units of penicillin.

Our own men in the next ward thought it all a huge joke. 'Give 'em your shoes to polish, Sister. They'll love it.'

A strange and moving situation occurred one day. One of the young German boys tentatively started up a song, while his comrades waited nervously to see how it would be received before joining in. We had no seriously ill men in the ward at that time; the boy had a pleasant voice, and we realised how long it had been since we heard anyone sing. We did nothing to discourage him. It was the catchy German marching song, 'Lili Marlene', which had become as popular with Monty's troops in Normandy as in Rommel's African campaign where it originated. The rest of the P.O.W.s, emboldened, now took up the song, singing in well-rehearsed harmonies that were a joy to hear. Then the moment enlarged to provide one of those memories that stay forever. From the adjacent British ward came the same song, sung in English. The surprised Germans responded to the compliment with even more enthusiastic singing, and Soutie and I stood between the two wards listening to a performance that would have done justice to a male voice choir from men who, until recently, had been doing their level best to kill each other.

'Just shows how daft war is,' said Soutie disgustedly.

I wondered if the same situation could have come about had the rôles of captor and captive been reversed?

Russell Slater was still doing the Dover-Arromanches run as M.O. on board an L.S.T. (Landing Ship, Tanks). These were wide vessels of a hollow design used for the bulk transport of tanks and troops. The flat bottom allowed the vessel to come close in-shore and a swing-down stern plating provided the necessary ramp for the speedy discharge of its cargo. Knowing that I was in the area, he had kindly dropped off a pound of coffee for me at the Beach Group in Arromanches. A message came to the hospital along with instructions for the next sea evacuations. '. . . and will Sister McBryde come to Beach Group 34 to pick up a packet of coffee.'

I persuaded Duff to accompany me and, greatly intrigued, we set off on our next free evening along the dusty road that led to the harbour and took up position to hitch a lift.

There was, as yet, no organised transport in Normandy, either civilian or military, but lifts were easy to come by. Since it was the only operational port, Cherbourg still not having been repaired after the long battle for its possession, transport went to and from Arromanches all day long.

The countryside around us was peaceful now. Lush summer growth had thrown a green wash over Normandy's scars. Cow parsley and rank weeds screened the burnt-out tanks in the ditches and the guns were miles away, somewhere near Arras. This was a peaceful backwater now.

We had not waited long before a jeep screeched to a halt in front of us. Three black American G.I.s beamed down at us. After a moment of indecision, I climbed into the back seat between two servicemen and Duff, in a loaded silence, took the seat next to the driver.

For some reason, the Americans were in a very uninhibited mood and seemed to find the situation vastly amusing, falling about with laughter, loose-limbed, wide-mouthed. Laughing childishly over the wheel, the driver put the vehicle in gear and we took off at a terrifying rate with Duff and me trying to smother our alarm and act as if this were a perfectly normal situation.

'Hole tight, Lootenant!'

In the back, I had nothing to hold tight to and rocked uncontrollably from one happy fellow to the other. Trees flew dizzily past and our course was wildly erratic.

'Where are you stationed, Sergeant?' I gasped, trying to cool the situation but this only increased their hilarity. The driver was laughing so hard that tears ran down his cheek as he cornered at great speed, handling the wheel with terrifying negligence.

Everything became clear when he reached down by the side of the driving seat and brought up a half-empty bottle of cognac.

'Have a swig, Lootenant.' He offered it to Duff with a flourish and no eyes at all on the road.

A look of alarm passed between Duff and myself. Enough was enough. I had not been leader of the Chaffinch Patrol for nothing! 'Stop at once, Corporal! You're drunk.' It was my Girl Guide's voice and there was no mistaking its pedigree. The grin on the driver's face wavered and we nearly went into the ditch as he turned to his companions for support.

'You're not fit to drive,' said Duff, looking like Queen Alexandra herself. 'Put us down at once.'

Sheepishly, he applied the brakes. After all, we had two pips up. The vehicle stopped, and thankfully we clambered out amid apprehensive silence.

Not till they were on their way again did they recover their bravado.

'Have yo'selves a ball!' was the last we heard as they went careering around the corner.

'Are you sure you want to go on with this?' Duff asked carefully.

'Of course,' I said confidently. 'It's just a question of getting the right lift.' I was determined to get my coffee.

The harbour looked vastly different from the night almost eight weeks ago when we were dropped at the end of the pier. The debris of battle had been cleared away and the beach was sectioned off into specific receiving areas. It had all the appearances of a busy, well-run port.

As Duff and I clambered down the dunes, an L.S.T. moved slowly out to sea on the turning tide, leaving its discharged cargo of trucks, tanks and supplies on the beach. Troops were loading up heavy transports and truck drivers prepared to move off.

'That looks like the chap we want to see,' Duff pointed to an officer in a battered R.E. cap and shirt sleeves who seemed to be in charge of operations on the beach. Major 'Robin' Hood R.E. and his staff, with liaison R.A.F. and R.N. officers, were responsible for the smooth running of what was the only working port in liberated France at that time. It was to remain so for some months to come.

He saw us as he made to return to the tumbledown beach H.Q. and called over, 'Come for the coffee? Come right in.'

The 34 Beach Group had set up their headquarters here in the remains of a shipwrecked vessel in the dunes on D-Day. A shacked-up extension of sorts had been added and it had taken on a look of permanency with tide-tables posted up and the C.O.'s name on the door. Inside the hotch-potch of tarpaulin and timber the men had made themselves comfortable. Sundry easy chairs and a fine red carpet had been 'requisitioned'. Photographs of the many ships that had used the port since

D-Day covered the rough planked walls. Capt. 'Fossy' Foster, the Major's second in command, put away his ledgers and opened the bar.

Duff and I, who had learned to be wary of situations like this in Normandy, gradually discarded our early warning systems and relaxed. Here were just two nice, happily married men, glad of some company, pleased to tickle our palate with a bottle of Champagne and a tin of salmon, and to pass around their family photographs. Surgeon Lt. Slater, they told us, had been in port the previous day and had left a bag of freshly roasted coffee with instructions to see that I got it.

'Next time he comes,' promised Robin, 'we'll take you out to his ship in a D.U.K.W. He never has time to come ashore.'

The other members of the Beach Group were coming in now, waiting their turn for a shower. 'Of course we've got a shower. We're Engineers, aren't we?' they said.

It was a rough and ready arrangement with a floor of sand but it did deluge one with cascades of hot water.

'And you must feel free to come and use it whenever you feel like it,' said Robin. 'Find your own way here and you can depend on us to get you back.'

It was 'Fossy' who took us home that night and, before the month was out, this group of benevolent Engineers was providing showers and hospitality for half the Sisters' Mess. And they did take me out in a D.U.K.W. the next time Russell's ship came in. I had pink gin and caviare in the Wardroom and a birthday cake two months early.

'You chose the wrong service, my girl,' said Surgeon-Lt. Slater, quite glorious in navy and gold.

10

A Trip to Rouen

By the end of August, we were pushing the Germans towards Belgium. Paris was French once more and now, at last, we could be sure that we would not be pushed back into the sea, which could foreseeably have happened at many stages during the last two months. Now we had Hitler on the run and this time there would be no Dunkirk.

We were able to arrange a day off a week. The question was, what to do with it? Soutie loved shopping. It was she who suggested a trip to Rouen.

'My orderly's just been. The shops are fabulous and dirt cheap because the Americans haven't been there.'

Pin held back. 'Are you sure that the Germans aren't still there?'

But the Germans were fleeing towards Belgium with Lt. General Horrocks and XXX Corps hard on their heels.

'They were chased out of Rouen days ago,' Soutie assured us. 'I've spent hardly a thing since I left England. Let's go.'

The next day, we walked to the newly constructed supply road that led from Arromanches to all points forward and chose a good position for hitching a lift.

Duff bent to my ear. 'Don't pick a drunk this time.'

'What's that about?' said Pin with a flash of suspicion.

'Here's a truck,' said Soutie. 'On your marks.'

The three-tonner was taking troops back to their units after a rest spell in Bayeux and willing hands helped us over the tailboard. (One of the first things you learned to do in Normandy was to climb decently into a truck whilst wearing a skirt.) The men were going beyond Rouen so we were assured of a lift all the way. Nothing could have been simpler.

As the road rolled away behind us, I recognised a familiar landscape. This was the way to Caen and, incredibly, here was the long line of refugees once more, only this time trudging in reverse, returning to see what, if anything, was left of their homes. The same old women in black and old men in berets, pushing the same handcarts, were going back to heaps of rubble. Soon we were lurching over mounds of bricks and mortar and we knew we had arrived in Caen. Huge blocks of the famous Caen stone had been thrown about haphazardly like sugar cubes. There was no telling where the original roads had been. William the Conqueror's city had been quite destroyed. Dark entrances like ratholes in the rubble showed where the returning civilians were living and a few makeshift shops were selling food. Any glances that came our way were understandably bitter. It was noon before we crossed the Seine at Rouen and the truck put us down by the damaged cathedral, leaning on its scaffolding like an elegant cripple.

But the town had got off lightly in the shelling and that afternoon we forgot about the war. Dark little shops selling handwrought silver jewellery, pure silk lingerie and French perfume drew francs from our wallets like magic. We rounded the day off with coffee and éclairs filled with real cream, a luxury long-since forgotten in England. Then it was time for the return journey.

The gendarme on the bridge regarded us in some astonishment.

'Mam'selle is not serious?' Nothing, he declared, went in that direction nowadays, except an occasional early morning truck. Everything was streaming into Belgium on a one-way trip that would end in Berlin.

'How did your orderly get back?' we demanded of Soutie and somewhat shamefacedly, she remembered that he had hospital transport to pick up medical equipment.

'Now she tells us,' groaned Duff.

With a Gallic shrug, the gendarme fell to picking his teeth again and we left him sitting in his sentry box and crossed to the other side of the bridge to consider our position. After an hour, during which time two jeeps and a farmcart went by in the opposite direction, Pin decided to have another go at the sentry.

'Look, Officer,' she said reasonably. 'We are nurses and we must be on duty in the morning in our hospital near Bayeux. Is there nothing you can do to help us?'

He spread his hands. 'Mam'selle, if a car would come, I would stop it, but I cannot make it come.' Irrefutable French logic.

The sun was setting behind the old, tiled roof-tops of the town. Lamps glowed in basement kitchens. It was the hour of food preparation. The heady smell of garlic sizzling in butter came sidling out from the narrow streets, and the gendarme came out of his box, locking the door behind him. Time for a pastis at Le Café au Coin. He pocketed the key and touched his cap to us.

'There's a good hotel in the town. Goodnight, Mam'selles.'

Our shopping trip was beginning to look like somebody's very stupid idea. We had about ninety miles to cover and no visible way of doing it except on our own two feet.

At that moment, unbelievably, a bright blue battered van chugged out of the town and creaked over the bridge towards us. A local fruiterer was on his way home after shutting up his shop in the town. When the situation was explained to him by the gendarme, he was courtesy itself. Whipping off his beret and bowing low, he held open the back of his small van and we climbed in beside the rotting pumpkins and squashed peaches.

'Is he going to Caen?' we pestered the gendarme who had had enough of us by this time.

'Oui!' said the gendarme excitedly, desperate for his pastis.

'Caen!' squealed the fruiterer in horror. 'Non, non!'

'Oh my God.' Soutie and I crawled out of the van again.

A furious conversation between the fruiterer and the gendarme ended abruptly in agreement and they turned to us, all smiles.

'Not quite into Caen,' explained the gendarme. 'But he will be pleased to take you as far as his house. It will be part of the way.' He said this with finality and set off determinedly for Le Café au Coin, having resolved the troublesome affair entirely to his satisfaction.

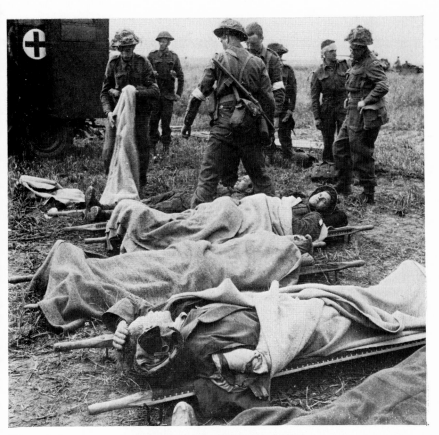

Wounded troops
being evacuated
from the
battlefield to a
Casualty
Clearing Station,
Normandy,
June 1944

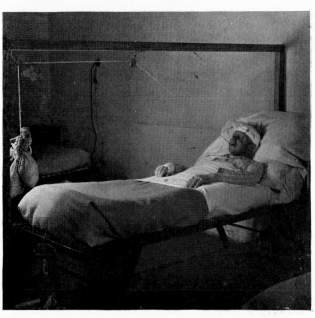

Soldier released
from P.O.W.
camp
undergoing
corrective
traction of the
jaw, Celle, June
1945

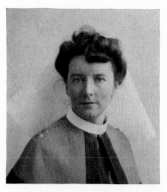

The author,
1945

Belsen, 1945,
shortly after the
arrival of the
Allies

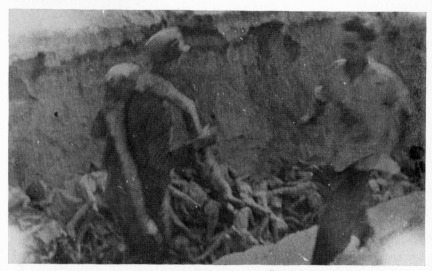

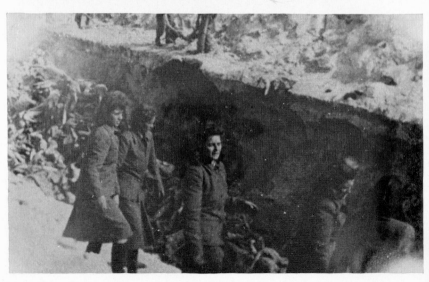

We gave Pin the front seat and the rest of us crawled into the back, necks bent to the low roof.

'En avant!' our driver cried gaily, with the air of one pulling away the chocks from an impatient flying machine, and we began to move forward in a series of jerks at a disappointing five miles an hour. 'Ho, ho!' he says archly, 'Very heavy ladies behind.' With every bump, we in the back were thrown about like a sack of potatoes.

'If it's going to be like this all the way to Caen, it'll be murder!' But we had barely gone six kilometres out of Rouen when we left the main road and took a very minor track through a dark wood. A short cut, we reassured ourselves. Instead, the van stopped outside a lonely cottage set amongst crowding trees. A light twinkled at a downstairs window and a chained dog set up a fearsome baying. Stunned by doubts, we made no move and eventually the fruiterer had to spell it out. This was his house and would we please get out of his van. He was late for dinner again, but there, he just had to help lame dogs over stiles. We could smell his dinner as he bade us goodnight and left us standing in the darkening forest.

Our tempers were frayed, our parcels a bore, companies of bats swept eerily over our heads, and roundly we cursed that fruit man as we stumbled back to the main road. The signpost, when we reached it, said Bayeux 145 km.

Pin was very quiet. Left alone, she would never have got herself into a scrape like this. We were a thoroughly bad influence on her. We set off to walk down the road, to walk to Bayeux, with a bright moon to light the way. The time was half-past ten. How fast must four nurses walk in order to cover 145 km by morning? I was about to suggest a running trot – with all these parcels? – when there was the welcome sound of a car coming up behind us. Arcs of light swung over the treetops from the headlights of a powerful vehicle, and a staff car braked to a standstill. We had made a human chain barrier and nothing could have got past without knocking us down.

It was a lieutenant of the Coldstream Guards returning from a mission to forward H.Q. and he was delighted to give us a lift, but not to Bayeux. His Mess was only a few miles down the road, in a very comfortable chateau, where, he assured us, there were plenty of beds. The Germans had left some excellent wine and it was time the boys had a party. But it was no good. We had to get to Bayeux, so regretfully, he handed us over to the Military Policeman at the next guard point, a broken down old Inn at a crossroads, l'Auberge du Roi. In the one undamaged room, an M.P. sat at an empty bar, reading a comic by the light of a Tilly lamp. His face showed complete disbelief as we piled out of the staff car.

'These ladies want a lift to Bayeux, Corporal.'

'Oh yes, sir?'

'Stop anything on four wheels going that way.'

'There'll be nothing going that way,' he said flatly. 'Not till the N.A.A.F.I. truck in the morning.'

'Goodbye, girls,' the lieutenant turned the car round. 'Sorry about the party.' He roared off, back to his Mess and his comfortable bed.

The dazed M.P. took us to the bar and pulled up some empty ammo boxes for seats. A primus flared on the rosewood bar counter. 'I was just brewing up,' he said diffidently. 'Don't know if there'll be enough cups.'

Mesmerised by the corporal's display of pin-ups, we sat in silence, drinking cocoa and reflecting ruefully that four wards were going to be short of a sister in the morning. At one time, l'Auberge du Roi must have been a well-appointed little inn but now ragged electric wires snaked down from a once elegantly moulded ceiling. Empty shelves flanked a cracked mirror advertising Stella Artois beer. Remnants of curtain hung at broken windows and the four corners of the room were littered with empty cigarette packets. An owl hooted in the deep countryside.

Duff shivered. 'What a lonely place.'

The M.P. looked up from his comic. 'You should have seen it last week. Like Piccadilly Circus. Troops and ammo moving all night long and the wood over there full of Jerry snipers. Nothing on the road at night now.'

From time to time, we stepped outside and strained our ears for the sound of an engine but there were only the noises of farmyard and countryside to be heard and a faraway church striking the quarters.

Then, when we had almost given up hope, the faint but unmistakeable chug-chug of a motor made itself felt rather than heard and we rushed headlong to the roadside. Something was coming, but we could see nothing. Then, out of the darkness, a darker shape loomed, weaving cautiously towards us.

'No friggin' lights,' muttered the M.P. 'Bet it's a Froggie. Halt!' he bellowed in a commanding voice. An unidentifiable vehicle pulling a trailer lurched up and stopped with a shudder at the corporal's feet.

'Where's your lights?' he demanded.

Two sharp, ferretty faces, dead white under black berets, peered down from the driver's cab. They broke into delighted grins. 'Les Anglais! All the blessed saints be praised!'

'Where's your lights!' the corporal said again.

The Frenchmen jumped down, joined by an older man and a youth who had been travelling in the trailer.

'The lights do not go, Corporal.'

The corporal lifted the bonnet. 'I'll have a look-see,' and he flicked on his torch. 'Psst!' he said, sidelong to us. 'If they're going your way, do you want a lift?'

We nodded frantically, even without lights.

'Where are you making for?' he turned to the Frenchmen.

'Lisieux,' said the older man whom they called Henri.

Lisieux was about half way. Better than nothing.

'And then Marseilles,' said the young boy excitedly, black eyes sparkling. 'We have just fought the Battle of Paris.' He flung an affectionate arm around the older man. 'My friends and me. Now we go to tell everyone that Paris is French again. The Germans —' he flicked his finger and thumb derisively, 'finish. Kaput.'

I noticed for the first time that they all carried guns at their belts. Le Maquis. These men were members of the French underground movement whose exploits were legendary.

'Give credit where it's due,' the corporal was still tinkering under the bonnet. 'You did a good job in Paris. Now, these ladies want a lift. Can you oblige?'

They all bowed, very deeply, and said they were enchanted, which we readily believed. A strong beam of light suddenly leapt across the road and the corporal straightened his back.

'Bravo!' yelled the Frenchmen.

'These blokes might be good at blowing up bridges but they don't know much about mechanics.' The corporal closed the bonnet and hastily began wiping his hands as one of the Frenchmen produced a bottle of cognac.

'A toast to Paris.' Henri ostentatiously wiped the mouth of the bottle before handing it to Pin.

'To Paris,' she spluttered and passed it on. She was not good on bottles.

The corporal pulled back the sleeve of his jacket and consulted the five German watches ranged up his forearm. Five minutes to midnight. 'You been lucky,' he said. 'Better get aboard.'

We followed Henri and the boy, who was known as le Bébé, into the trailer while the other two Frenchmen climbed into the driving seat and started up the engine. Instantly, the contents of the trailer began to rattle and shake alarmingly. It had been home for these men for many months and was filled with the paraphenalia of living and fighting. A kettle swung over a pile of Sten guns, tin plates clattered in an enamel bowl. A small tin nailed to one of the side struts of the vehicle beneath a square of mirror held a precious sliver of soap. We settled ourselves on two mattresses spread over the floor amongst bundles of clothing and boxes of ammunition and watched the darkness swallow the last glimpse of l'Auberge du Roi.

We were the only people on the roads. The villages we passed through were full of sleep and shadows. Our lights picked out letters painted three feet high on orchard walls – 'Vive le Tommy!'. By the light of a hand torch the Frenchmen showed us photographs of the liberation of Paris.

'I killed as many Germans as I could,' le Bébé said proudly.

It was hard to believe he was a desperate insurgent. He looked such a boy.

The hours crept by and we dozed fitfully until around two in the morning when we were jerked awake by the truck stopping. We were in the courtyard of a farmhouse where lights burned in a downstairs window.

'Supper,' said Henri, and handed us down from the back of the trailer. Wearily we followed the men to where a woman now stood silhouetted in the open door of the house.

'We thought the Boche had got you.' She welcomed the men with a warm embrace, and looked curiously at us.

'Where are we?' I asked Henri.

'Lisieux,' he said. 'After supper, we will take you all the way to Bayeux.'

In a room beyond the kitchen, a cheerful fire burned beneath posters of General de Gaulle, General Eisenhower and Winston Churchill, and a dozen or so men and women seated at a central table sprang up with shouts of welcome for our friends. An old crone nodding by the fire jumped awake and a dog at her feet flagged its tail in greeting. We were led to seats at the table and thick tumblers were placed in front of us. 'Vive la France!' somebody called and filled our glasses with red wine.

'Tell about Paris, Henri.'

Henri lit his cigarette and blew out a cloud of smoke. He told of the beginning, the insurrection of the loyal French police, the rallying of the citizens. He described how barricades were put up in the streets. He showed pictures of the Quai d'Orsay blocked with burning tanks and then he came to the German capitulation. American forces had been on their way to help but the French were proud to have freed Paris themselves. 'We marched them through the streets, with their hands above their heads. That was a sight, my friends.'

We were as enthralled as the others, following as well as we could with our school French and when Henri gave the toast – 'To Paris. French once more' – we jumped up with the rest of them and emptied our glasses.

Now the toasts came thick and fast, de Gaulle, Eisenhower,

Churchill and finally, with many sidelong glances, *les Anglaises*. But *les Anglaises* were feeling decidedly woozy by this time, what with tiredness and the wine and nothing to eat since those memorable éclairs, and when someone squeezed my knee under the table I found it impossible to guess who, amongst all these uproariously happy Frenchmen, was the culprit.

They were all ordinary people around that table, farmers, clerks, housewives and shop assistants who, by fate, had been turned into saboteurs and spies, experts in explosives, cartography and decoding. The wireless set had not always sat so boldly in the centre of the table nor, during the Occupation, had the door been left unguarded. Tonight they were celebrating freedom.

Bread and plates of meat and soft discs of delicious cheese were brought out and it was almost four o'clock before Henri signalled to us. 'Mam'selles. Bayeux.'

Miserably we realised that it was on our account that the party was breaking up but they insisted that Bayeux was *en route* for Marseilles and we were in no state to argue. Henri took the wheel and Michel, who had been driving, joined us in the back with le Bébé. In five minutes we were dead asleep, all jostled up together on the mattresses. I awakened to daylight and le Bébé shaking us by the shoulders.

'There are hospitals all the way,' he complained. 'Which one is yours?'

Outside the 75th, having no wish to draw attention to ourselves, we said goodbye as discreetly as possible. They kissed our grubby hands and drove away in a truck which, by daylight, looked utterly dilapidated. We marvelled that we had made the journey without mishap in such a wreck and stood waving until it rattled out of sight.

'Next time we go shopping,' said Pin tersely, 'let's try somewhere a little nearer.'

We hurried into the hospital field. The night staff were bent over their reports and a spiral of smoke rose from the cookhouse. There was just time to change, grab a quick cup of coffee and, incredibly, we would be on duty in time.

'What's up with you, Sister?' asked one of my patients as I yawned over his temperature chart. 'Been out on the tiles all night?'

It was Sunday morning. The padres in their dining-tents-converted-into-chapels were preparing the Sacrament and Normandy churches filled with people eager to give thanks for deliverance from war. It was 3rd September, five years to the day since Britain had declared war on Germany.

11

The Advance to Brussels

The hot and bloody summer was over in Normandy. Ours was now one of the last hospitals on 'Harley Street'. The war had gone far beyond us and most of the other hospitals had moved further up the line. A wildly enthusiastic Brussels had greeted the Welsh and Grenadier Guards on 3rd September as they entered a city hastily abandoned by the Germans. At the same time, American troops were racing from the Meuse to the Moselle. The Germans were having a taste of their own 'blitzkrieg'.

I was back on Resus., this time on night-duty and on my own for it was rare for us to receive a casualty in a state of shock these days. Convoys of wounded were intercepted by hospitals further up the line. This night, no patients awaited me. The trestles were bare. The tarpaulin floor was newly swept and the desk-top neat and tidy. I intended to help on the wards after a routine check of equipment. Then Major MacPherson, still in operating gown, came in from the annexe. There were two badly injured P.O.W.s about to leave the theatre and he suggested that, since I had no other patients, they should come back to Resus. instead of proceeding to the wards.

'One of them is in very poor shape,' he said. 'Not much chance of his lasting the night.'

He was about twenty-two years old and had lost almost the whole of one shoulder with a shell. Even now, after an extensive cleaning-up operation, there was deep, uncontrollable bleeding and his blood pressure was steadily sinking. The other German, a red-haired young man who had lost a foot and an arm, seemed to be stabilising, and settled into a restful sleep.

Major Mac., helping me to make the badly injured youth comfortable on pillows as he came round from the anaesthetic, looked down on the drawn, white face. He slowly shook his head. 'Come for me if you need me. I'll be in my bunk.'

In the night that followed I stayed by the side of the desperately wounded man. There was no-one else to claim my time. I checked pulse and blood pressure, monitored transfusions, moistened his dry lips. His head tossed impatiently with the restlessness that tells of haemorrhage and his eyes ranged unseeing around the tent. Once or twice, they fixed on me, pale lashes blinking with concentration. I spoke to him, in my bad German, hoping that it might help him to know he was not alone in his battle.

I did not need to send for Major Mac. A small miracle was worked through the night. Those bleeding vessels which were too deep to suture, sealed of their own accord. I realised what was happening when slowly but surely his blood pressure began to rise and his restless head lay still for the space of a short, light sleep that took the frown from his sweating forehead. The dark blue night at the squared window in the tentside gave way to a pale grey. He had survived the worst night of his life. I held a feeding cup of water while he drank eagerly and there was intelligence in his eyes now as he looked at me and at my uniform.

'Danke,' he said, with an infinitesimal nod of his head. He was on the evacuation list a week later and probably never went without a shirt again for as long as he lived.

Mornings were chill now with long scarves of mist trailing at the edge of the wood where we camped. The grass in our field was worn bare in places and our tents were bleached by the sun, the wind and the rain. We felt that we had been left behind by the war. We had seen the Normandy orchards bloom with apple blossom and now it was harvest time. All around us, the routine of the seasons was smoothing away the disruptions of war. It was time to repair barns before the winter, to fill in shell-holes. Women and children heaped little carts with apples for the cider presses and farmers tended secret stills of Calvados.

We were back into A.V.s and gumboots once more for the floors of our tents were cold and muddy. Nights were growing chill and we wore football jerseys over our pyjamas and long, woollen operation stockings. The hospital no longer concentrated on surgery. We had a skin department now and medical wards. Our trade was in athlete's foot, cystitis and ingrowing toe nails, dull stuff indeed after our heroic beginning. The unit was bored. Army regulations were tightened up.

'Become very sloppy since we landed,' said the Colonel. 'Keep everyone on their toes.'

Army forms multiplied, patients' lockers once more resumed paramount importance and the latrines reeked of chloride of lime. An entertainments committee launched itself into a Christmas Pantomime, and a Brains Trust argued its way through every Tuesday night. Captain Franklin, the skin specialist, and Captain Merivale, pathologist, stole away each evening to practise Bach fugues on clarinet and flute in the mortuary, while the less talented amongst us haunted the barn of an enterprising farmer near by where, for a few francs, we could buy a bowl of rough cider and talk about all the wonderful things we would do after the war was over. It was a hang-fire time of disinclination and apathy. Even E.N.S.A. had moved up the line. There was the occasional Company dance enlivened by Lt. Colonel Murray of our Medical Division who invariably lost his temper when we made a mess of the eightsome reel, as we always did, and there were many parties. We were satiated with parties. American messes in the area were particularly generous. They provided music for dancing and superb food but bored and lonely soldiers far from home are sometimes difficult to handle. More and more, we preferred to stay within our own camp.

The prospect of winter in Normandy seemed bleak. We were sick of mud for a bedroom carpet, sick of bathing in a tin box, sick of having nowhere to hang our clothes. This bout of self-pity was cut short by the arrival of Pioneers to put up Nissen huts in place of the tents. At last we had a real bathroom with hot showers and a place to do our ironing, a place to wash hair, and a cast-iron stove that glowed red-hot in the middle of each hut.

We barely had time to relish this luxury when the order came to move. The 75th was to do a 250 mile hop to Belgium, from the mud of Normandy to the sophistication of Brussels. Our morale soared and we gladly handed over our patients to a unit fresh from England.

'Nissen huts! My dear, how ghastly!'

On a cold, grey morning in November, the 75th convoy prepared to leave. From where we sat in the back of a three-tonner, squashed together for warmth under a tarpaulin, we could see unfamiliar sisters moving in and out of our wards, coming to terms with the mud, teetering nicely across the duckboards, and we looked for the last time on the field that had seen so much trauma. Our Hospital Office produced some remarkable statistics. Since that opening day at the beginning of July, 7579 casualties had been admitted. During the first four weeks, 4535 had been evacuated to Britain, another 1000 had been discharged to their units. 205 men had died. The recovery rates of all men wounded in Normandy was good.* Ninety-three per cent of all those who reached medical units recovered. We felt justifiably proud of the part our hospital had played.

Through Amiens and Arras, Passchendaele and Mons we drove, and across the plains of Picardy where, thirty years earlier, putteed legs had marched to 'Tipperary' and 'Pack up your Troubles'. In the early evening we entered the sprawling suburbs of Brussels.

Of all the cities liberated by the Allies, none was so enthusiastic in its welcome as Brussels. Even now, two months after the Guards' triumphal entry, we were given a great reception. People in the street, complete strangers, came up to shake us by the hand. Old ladies embraced us with tears in their eyes. We were given hospitality at all levels and there were many levels in Brussels. It was a city of contrasts. Elegant shops displayed lingerie of crêpe-de-chine and chic coats of rabbit fur, yet old folk armed with hatchets crept out as soon as darkness fell to chop down hoardings for firewood when the gendarme was not looking.

Soutie and I were passing by the Public Library one day when one of the librarians hurried down the steps towards us, a slight, elderly lady at her side. The librarian handed us a

* 21st Army Group Statistics.

visiting card by way of introducing her companion. Madame, who did not speak much English, would be very happy if we would visit her the following week in the afternoon.

On the day, we took a tram for the address was a little way out of town. All transport was free for Allied troops, consequently the trams were overcrowded. There was barely room for a foothold on the outer steps for Soutie and me. We hung on to the belt of an unknown passenger who had a firm grip on a door handle somewhere within, and hoped for the best.

Madame lived in a street of houses that had seen better days, with heavily-curtained sitting-rooms on the first floor and dark basements. Only the basements were lived in now. With coal at its exorbitant price, she explained, heating the whole house was out of the question. We followed her along a gloomy passage and down the stairs to where the servants used to live. Her white haired husband was on his feet to welcome us into what had become their living-room. Comfortable furniture had been moved down here, easy chairs and a round table with maroon tasselled cover, but the only form of heating was a gas ring on an ancient stove. We were given rugs to put over our knees and we did not remove our great coats as we sat and talked to these two kindly old people who made us as welcome as if we had been their daughters.

Madame fussed happily over a pan of milk at the stove while her husband told us the story of the liberation of Brussels. After the sudden flight of the Germans, citizens from the poorer parts had raided the Town Hall, carrying away in wheelbarrows the stolen wine hoarded there by the occupying troops. There was no-one to hinder them for the city was temporarily without government or the forces of law and order. There was a good deal of drunken rejoicing in some quarters but most of the city waited apprehensively through the rest of that unreal day, 2nd September. The next day, British tanks came rolling through the streets and British Tommies, dead beat after their headlong rush across country, bivouacked on the boulevards in the heart of a city gone quite mad with gratitude.

Madame served hot chocolate in pretty little cups which she

handed to Soutie and me with one of the few English phrases she knew: 'Thank you, Tommie.'

A different kind of invitation came one day for Duff, Margaret Fairy and myself as we dawdled over a shop counter. Two attractive women elegantly wrapped in fur and wearing outlandish creations on their heads, invited us to dine with them. They lived in the smart part of town in a block of apartments comfortably warmed by a coal-fired central-heating boiler. We joined a sophisticated company of men and women in evening dress around a table sparkling with crystal and silver. Alongside these beautifully dressed women, we felt awkwardly out of place in uniform but they heaped kindness and attention on us. The food was superb and dinner lasted for most of the evening with breaks for conversation and dancing. There were no shortages of any kind here, yet not so far away, in the poorer quarter we had seen trespassing urchins throw down handfuls of coal from the delivery trucks to their furtive, scrambling mothers below.

We were billetted in a block of flats designed for old people and we revelled in the luxury. There were wardrobes for our clothes and dressing tables with mirrors. Our weatherbeaten faces seemed strangely out of place in these civilised surroundings. We rushed to the hairdressers to be permed and groomed. Gumboots went down to the bottom of the trunks once more, along with A.V.s, and we sent our grey suits to the cleaners. Brussels was a lively city with plenty for us to do in our off-duty time. A favourite spot was the Officers' Club at the Plaza in the Boulevarde Adolphe Max, with a dance floor the size of a postage stamp, a string quartet and a bottle of Château d'Yquem waiting at a candlelit table. It was just what we wanted after the doldrums of Normandy.

The hospital building was an ex-clothing factory used by the Germans for the manufacture of uniforms for the Wehrmacht and there were mountains of buttons and coat-hangers to be cleared away before we could set up the beds. The rooms were suitably large and light and there were cupboards to hold our medicines and equipment, a great convenience after the Compo boxes of Normandy. There were no draughts whistling through

tent flaps and no need to hump jerrycans about. There was
running water. Hot drinks could be quickly made on a gas ring.

Our first casualties were Canadians who had been given the
unenviable task of winkling out Germans from heavily fortified
positions in the Scheldt estuary. Casualties were high and we
were back to major surgery again. Although Antwerp had been
taken on the 4th September, the much needed port could not
be put into operation because of enemy guns commanding the
estuary. This lack of any suitable port other than Arromanches
for the landing of supplies was seriously slowing down the
Allied advance and foul November weather now added a
further complication. Even tracked vehicles became bogged
down in the unceasing rain. The impetus of British and American
troops was brought to a halt in the flooded lowlands of the
rivers Maas and Roer.

In Brussels we were not aware of this. Preparations for the first
liberated Christmas were in hand and we delighted in the
decorated streets and shop windows. Nine days before Christmas, snow began to fall completing the storybook illusion.
Then the shattering news burst upon us that the Germans had
made a strong counter-attack in the region of the Ardennes and
that they were advancing at a great rate with new Panzer
divisions formed at miraculously short notice. They were head-
ing for Antwerp in an attempt to drive a wedge between the
Allies and force them back on to the flooded rivers.

It was a cruel turn of Fate for the people of Brussels. There
was panic as those who could leave packed their bags and fled.
Those who could not leave, took down their Allied flags, closed
their doors and waited.

On Christmas Eve, with the advancing Germans only sixty
miles from Brussels, I went with Duff to midnight Mass at the
great cathedral of St. Gudule. A silent, heavy-hearted crowd
was making its way over snow-covered pavements to pray
together for deliverance. Many Allied uniforms mingled with
the local people. The deliverance that we prayed for came on
two counts. Hitler ran out of petrol and the weather changed,
allowing air support for our hard-pressed troops.

New Year celebrations also failed to come up to expectations as far as my friends and I were concerned. The Scots contingent had planned a fine old Hogmanay and Soutie, Pin, Duff and I joined them on our return from a celebratory dinner at the Services Club which had misfired badly when we realised that the waiters had embarked on a little private profiteering. 'And Bonne Année to you too,' I said crossly as I picked up our minute change. Much in need of good cheer, we joined Andy and Janet Smart in a bedroom packed with Scottish Q.A.s, to find Janet sobbing her way through 'It's aye that I'm longing for my ain folk', and Andy dropping tears into her whisky.

There was no time for a hangover the next morning. We awakened to alarms and the sound of machine-gunning. B 56 airfield at nearby Evère was being strafed by enemy raiders. These New Year greetings from the Germans were their last attack in the vicinity of Brussels, although they continued to fight in the Ardennes until 8th January when their offensive finally petered out.

Soon we were to be given the opportunity of seeing 'our ain folk' back home. First allocations of leave were beginning to come through and three or four of us at a time were flown from Brussels for a welcome two weeks' leave. This was our first trip home since D-Day plus thirteen, a lifetime of experience away. To our eyes, accustomed as we were to war-torn Europe, England seemed unbelievably green and unspoilt as we approached by air.

When we had time to look about us in the streets, we were struck by the confident bearing of passers-by. Tradesmen and housewives alike seemed different beings from the war-weary civilians of the days before the Second Front. Owners of city houses were returning to their boarded-up homes, in spite of Hitler's V-2 bombs. My home town of Whitley Bay was full of bustle once again though many shop windows were without glass and bomb-damaged houses not yet repaired. I dressed in mufti once more and became anonymous in cinema queues.

Bellingham, the grey stone village on the North Tyne where my sister lived, seemed unaltered except that there were few

young men around on Mart Day. Their fathers did the shep-
herding in the stockyards now. The local schoolmaster and one
of the bank manager's sons were prisoners of war and a handful
of new names would be added to the war memorial that stood in
the High Street.

In London, I looked up my friend, Helen Armstrong, the
art student who had started life in the W.A.A.F.s as an assistant
cook. She was now a Flight Officer involved in top secret activities at the Air Ministry. Good-looking and impeccably uniformed, she waited for me on the steps of Swan and Edgar in
Piccadilly. I arrived to find her usual composure considerably
shaken. She had just been nudged out of her position by a
prostitute and told to find her own beat. The next day, I
reported to Northolt to take the plane back to Brussels.

12

No. 5 Maxillo-Facial Unit

Soon after my return from leave, on my way out of the 'ladies' one night at the club in the Boulevarde Adolphe Max, I came face to face with Lieut. Wigglesworth and his friend, Captain Fuller. I had last seen 'Wiggy' in our Normandy hospital visiting one of his men who had been badly wounded. When he introduced me to his friend I had some difficulty in shaking hands as I was carrying a hatful of eggs. The club lavatory attendant ran a few hens in her Brussels' back-yard and we had an arrangement to swop my N.A.A.F.I. chocolate with her eggs. Now that we had kitchen facilities, some of us liked to experiment with cooking.

'I must have a look in the "Gents",' said Pat Fuller soberly. 'See what I can find.'

His unit, Movement Control, was based in Shell Mex Buildings, Brussels, and the next few days saw us wining and dining together whenever I had an evening off duty.

'What's this Movements man like?' Pin asked curiously as I hurried to keep an appointment.

I stopped and considered. 'He's got the kindest eyes you ever saw,' I said.

Pin sniffed. 'I suppose all the others were brutes.'

Towards the middle of January, Pin and I were posted. On the strength of our plastic surgery experience in Bangour, we were sent to the 108th B.G.H. which occupied a modern civilian hospital in the centre of the city and was host at the present time to No. 5 Maxillo-Facial Unit. These units were small and very mobile, dealing entirely with facial injuries. In the 1914–18 war, this category of wounded had been given low priority, and the resultant mortality from shock, to which these casualties are especially prone, was very high indeed. The revised approach was to get them to medical treatment without delay, a step which brought about an immediate rise in recovery rates.

The Maxillo-Facial units, nicknamed 'Max Factors', functioned independently, attaching themselves to whichever medical unit was near the fighting for the purpose of sharing such facilities as light, water, power, sewerage and sterilising equipment. At the time of our posting, there was a whole ward at the 108th B.G.H. given over to facially injured men and our minds went back to the pedicles and grafts of Bangour. But here in Brussels we were at the other end of the chain of treatment. There was no question of grafting at this stage. The men we were to nurse had just been injured. The job on hand was to clean up the damage in order to produce a healthy field for the reconstructive surgery which would come later in hospitals at Park Prewitt, East Grinstead and Bangour.

Pin and I were sad to leave our friends at the 75th but we were still able to meet in off-duty time and we were eager to involve ourselves once more in facial surgery. The two surgeons, Major Fitzgibbon, C.O. of the unit, and Capt. Tommy Gibson, assisted by dental surgeons Major Holland and Major Irwin, dealt with all fractured jaws and other facial injuries in this area of the front, painstakingly patching together whatever could be saved of a man's face. It was our job in the ward to see that these stichlines were kept free from sepsis and that the patients' strength was maintained by any one of several methods of feeding. Lunchtime was a performance calling for maximum patience on the part of the nurse and the recipient. There were men with splinted jaws where a little gap had been made by the extraction of two front teeth to allow the passage of a teaspoonful of mince. For others lunch was liquid, coming down a funnel and tube, but in every case it had to be adequate and rich in the vitamins necessary to speed the healing processes.

'Mind you clean that pudding off my sewing, hen.' Redhaired Tommy Gibson from Glasgow watched me as I carefully spooned rice pudding into the mouth of a lieutenant who had a large hole in one cheek. To the intense frustration of the patient, who was hungry, a great deal of the food found its way out through the hole and I had to direct the teaspoon with care to make sure that some of the pudding went down the right way. Tommy's tiny, black silk stitches traversed the inside of the man's mouth like lines on a road map. These had to be scrupulously cleaned by gentle irrigation with a syringe after each meal.

The lieutenant had led an attack over a bridge he knew to be mined. Some men had to be sacrificed in an advance. Now the war was over for this brave man. The injury to his cheek was the least of his worries. He was blinded, whether temporarily or not it was hard to say at this stage, and he had lost a leg. He asked me to write a note to his wife to say that he was surviving.

There was suddenly an excess of spit and polish when the news came that General Montgomery was to pay a visit to the hospital. Timetables for treatments and dressings were altered so that 'Monty' would find the wards neat and tidy, all orderlies in clean, white smocks and Q.A.s in impeccable uniform. But delays in dressings and irrigations would have been uncomfortable and detrimental to our Maxillo-Facial patients and I went about my business in the usual way, trusting that I had some immunity from the rules of the 108th B.G.H. As a result, when the General did his tour of the wards, I was busy with a dressing trolley, the only sister in mask and gown. To my surprise and delight, he passed by the respectful groups of Q.A.s waiting to welcome him and strode to where I stood with my trolley by the side of a bed. Meeting the penetrating glance from his very blue eyes was like connecting with an electric current. His grin was frank and friendly.

'Don't let me hold you up, Sister.' He shook my hand in a grip that left the fingers tingling long after he had whirled away. Perhaps he, too, did not agree with V.I.P. treatment for hospital visitors.

The Sisters' Mess for the 108th was in the Hotel Regina, all lace curtains, rattling hot water radiators and pot plants. There were new faces for Pin and me to get to know and new culprits to pinch the *Daily Telegraph* crossword. But I was not to remain long with Pin, for when the 'Max Factors' moved on to Holland at the beginning of February, I was posted to join them as ward sister. There were two other sisters on the strength of the unit who were concerned mainly with the theatre. It was decided that a third sister to watch the ward would be useful. This was considered a better arrangement than the usual system of borrowing a sister, who was not trained in the work from the host hospital. It was all a matter of chance that I was posted instead of Pin and I was sorry to have to leave her now amongst comparative strangers at the 108th.

I sent a message to Shell-Mex Building and Pat Fuller and I had a last dinner together at the club. He had a friend on an airfield somewhere near Eindhoven, which was where I was going, and thought he might be able to get a lift in the Auster light aircraft that flew mail to the forward troops. I hoped that I would see him again.

The 'Max Factors' occupied a monastery on the outskirts of Eindhoven. My room was a bare little cell overlooking the monks' graveyard and furnished simply with a wooden cot and a chair. From the window, I had a view of the route taken by XXX Corps on its way to Arnhem in the ill-fated 'Market-Garden' operation. It was a straight and narrow road, wrecked vehicles clearly showing that its verges had been mined. Low-lying fields fell away on either side, striped with dark, drainage ditches brimful after recent rains. The ward given over to Maxillo-Facial surgery had been the monks' refectory and was a large, high-ceilinged room with dead-white walls and Gothic script trailing over its windows. The casualties were men who had been caught in the flooded lowlands of the Rhine and Maas, wounded within sight of Germany. To set foot at last on German soil would have been something to write home about but, bogged down with their vehicles, they were easy targets for German air attacks and they were lucky to be alive; burnt men with faces puffed up like balloons, men with windpipes blocked by injury to tongue or palate who could not breathe except through a tracheotomy (a surgical opening into the trachea), men in helmets of plaster of Paris sprouting steel rods screwed to splinted jaws.

These men were my responsibility and with them came

Thompson, a twenty-year-old clay processor from Stoke-on-Trent, who was my orderly. Thompson liked to wear plimsolls on duty and flicked noiselessly about his business in Will O'the Wisp bedside patterns, stripping beds in the twinkling of an eye, shaving, bathing and feeding the men with never so much as the clink of a teaspoon or the clash of a dish. It was a quiet, calm place and the monks would not have been disturbed to see how their premises were used.

This feeling of serenity originated in the operating theatre. Major Fitzgibbon and Capt. Gibson operated there in an air of complete tranquillity. I never saw the Major ruffled and Tommy Gibson's ginger eyelashes would bat away for hours above his green mask as he manipulated small, curved suture needles with never a touch of clumsiness or hint of impatience. These two, with Major Thornton the anaesthetist and two first-class theatre sisters, Sister Olivia Holmes and Sister Vaughan-Jones, worked together to transform the dirty, pulpy mass left by shell explosion into a clean area where what remained of the structures of the face could be repaired. Torn blood vessels were sutured. Edges of tissue which could be approximated were stitched together again and the dirt of the battlefield was washed away.

The casualties themselves were uncomplaining beyond belief. Propped up on their pillows, bandaged and splinted, they followed my progress with their eyes as I pushed my dressing trolley from one bed to the next. Those who were unable to speak, like the Guardsman who was being kept alive on eggnogs poured down his nasal tube, would hand me little notes.

'Steak and chips tonight, Sis? Or shall we try the Duck à l'Orange?'

In spite of all the tragedy, the ward was a happy place.

One day a sergeant of the 51st Highland Division was carried in, propped upright on a stretcher by rolled blankets. 'Let him fall back and he's a gonner,' the M.O. at the Regimental Aid Post had warned the bearers. A sodden dressing covered the lower half of his face and a piece of gauze fluttered over the tracheotomy at his throat. From his medical record card I learned that a flying hunk of mortar had carried his lower jaw clean away and an emergency tracheotomy had been carried out. Crouched in a ditch near the Rhine approaches, the M.O. saved the sergeant's life with a scalpel and an air tube and, with everything going up around him, sent him down the line to us.

After resuscitation, he was on the operating table for two and a half hours while the surgeons removed the earth and grit of the ditch and shreds of khaki cloth from the pulpy mess which was all that remained below the sergeant's top lip. They dug out cruel shell splinters and bits of shattered jaw bone, stitching together any skin edges that were left, in order to close the wound.

Thompson and I received him gently back to bed and watched him carefully through anaesthesia.

'Poor bugger,' murmured the tank commander in the next bed who could hardly see out of his swollen, burnt eyelids, and the men who could not speak made little grunts of sympathy.

When the time came for the sergeant's first post-operative dressing, I wheeled my trolley to his bedside where he sat, propped on pillows, only his bright, black eyes showing above the bandaged lower half of his face. As I moved his locker to make room for the trolley, my eye fell on a photograph there of a good-looking young soldier in Scottish dress with his arm about the waist of a smiling girl. The thought ran through my mind that if this was our sergeant, then his girl friend was in for a shock.

Carefully, I took down the outer dressings and, with forceps, removed the gauze packs from a tongue so swollen and stitched that it was barely recognizable. There was, of course, no lower framework to the face for the jaw had gone. I kept my expression blank for the sergeants' bright eyes were on me. Then I saw his gaze pass over my shoulder and rivet upon something there. Silently I cursed the chromium dressing drum on my trolley which was as good as a mirror, but it was too late to do anything about it so I went on cleansing the stitchlines and re-packing the tongue.

When I finished, he rested his head on the freshened pillows, his tracheotomy puffing more urgently after his exertion, and reached with an exploring hand for the pad and pencil always kept on the bed. My heart sank, for I could guess the nature of the question he would put, but when I took the note, it read, 'When's your night off, Gorgeous?'

When he saw me laugh, his eyes twinkled naughtily, like two little lights in a void, and I ticked him off, called him a Cheeky Charlie and he loved it. I felt inadequate in the face of such courage.

Then there was the endless patience of the bombardier with extensive burns to face and hands. His dressing took me an hour and must have been distressing but he never made the slightest murmur of complaint; rather, he was at pains to assist me in any way possible. He had lost the fleshy, external portions of his ears and nose, and his eyes were slits in a swollen bladder of a face. I had to swab most gently the whole area with saline solution, paying great care over the eyes and nostrils where crusty secretions formed. Then I dusted his face with sulphonamide powder and covered it with squares of sterile, vaselined net. A light mask cut out of sterilised cotton covered the whole. Bearing in mind those distorted hands of the Bangour pilot, I took great pains over his fingers, letting him float them in a bowl of warm saline and encouraging him to make as many movements as possible while they were immersed. They were then patted dry, dusted with sulphonamide powder and each finger separately wrapped in vaseline gauze. Finally, I rested the whole wrist and hand on a cock-up splint so that muscles and tendons could not contract. I hoped that he would be left with useful hands. I would never see the final results.

The ward was full of brave men like these. Had they always been stoics, I wondered? Or was it some divine compensation for their horrific disfigurement. And what about the girls in the photographs? Would they accept the boy friends and the husbands with new faces? If they did not, then these men would be casualties a second time.

13

Crossing the Rhine: Celle

Allied troops reached the Rhine at the beginning of March 1945. Germany's great river was desperately defended, and, although the Americans made a daring crossing over the Upper Rhine on 7th March, minutes before the last bridge was blown up, the wider reaches of the Lower Rhine were not in our hands until the end of the month. Here, not a bridge had been left standing by the retreating Germans. Between Duisburg and Coblenz alone, twelve bridges had been destroyed.

Once the Rhine was crossed, our unit was able to move forward. We had been at Eindhoven for almost a month during which time we had not seen much of the town, operating as we did on the outskirts. There had been little incentive for us to explore. Philips' extensive electronics factory had attracted considerable attention from air attacks and large areas were laid waste. Now, at the beginning of April, we dispatched our patients down the line and prepared to move on, packing of equipment being done by our very efficient O.R.A.s and dental technicians.

We were to rendezvous with our old friends, the 'Heads' unit, at the border town of Venlo, then proceed after an overnight stop into Germany as a combined unit of 'Heads and Faces'. Our joint accommodation for the night was in another monastery, smaller than the one we had just vacated and we sisters had to share beds. It was suggested that, for fairness, the largest should sleep with the smallest. Naturally, I was paired with Sister Bell of 'Heads' who was big, plump and bouncy, and consequently I hardly slept a wink in a wooden cot designed for one narrow monk.

I was not the only one to be upset by our travel arrangements. Major Holland, who was usually easy-going and affable, was in a thoroughly unsociable mood the next morning as we prepared to move into Germany.

'What's the matter with him?' pouted Sister Vaughan-Jones.

Olivia Holmes threw it off casually. 'He's just cross because his Bronco hasn't caught up with him.'

'Bronco?'

'Toilet paper. He has it sent from England. Doesn't like service issue.' Each of us had different priorities.

Once across the border, we saw how things were with the German civilians. The towns we passed through showed all the scars of recent street fighting: blasted steeples, roofless houses, and walls pock-marked with bullet holes. Shot-up vehicles had been abandoned by the roadside and one British ambulance had a shellhole right through its red cross.

Shocked civilians hung sheets and pillow-slips from the windows of their wrecked homes: the white flag of surrender and the no less white face of defeat. They had been promised the earth and domination over every other race and now they were watching the invasion of their proud Fatherland. Captured German infantry stumbled by on their way to the P.O.W. cages. Nothing was left but despair.

In order to clear up head and facial casualties which were in transit through the immediate area at that time, we opened up our unit for a brief stop of only a few days south-west of Wesel, the point at which British troops had crossed the Rhine a week earlier. We attached ourselves to a Casualty Clearing Station which had already established itself in a field next to an abandoned German factory, Schafers' Propellor Works, near enough to make use of its light, power and water. We unpacked and set up the theatres straight away and I joined the C.C.S. sisters in their ward tent where I was to look after 'Max-Factor' cases. A C.C.S., by its nature, was always in a forward position with a correspondingly heavy work load. Sister Walker, who was in charge of this particular C.C.S., was very deservedly decorated for her efficient management of this busy unit under sustained pressure.

We were under canvas again at the C.C.S. It was early April and fine weather for sleeping out of doors. A little dachshund, 'Fritzie', adopted us and his long wet nose ferretted us out of our bedrolls in the early mornings. But we had to move on after a few days in order to keep up with the rapidly advancing forward troops. Once over the Rhine, the front line had become very mobile with some points thrusting far ahead, leaving bewildered German units behind on the flanks. Our destination was a point sixty miles on the other side of the Rhine, a town called Wettringen near Rheine on the River Ems. We were to join up there with a 200-bed hospital which was also on its way at that moment.

On 7th April we crossed the Rhine by Bailey bridge at what was left of the once thriving commercial town of Wesel, now flattened by the carpet of bombs put down ahead of our attacking troops. The remains of its bridge dipped crazily into a river still high with spring floods. The devastation continued on the other side. Haggard civilians abandoned to their fate stood by their white sheets, while distant gunfire rumbled in the background. Our trucks made slow progress on roads congested with P.O.W.s, long columns of weary men with sometimes no more than one British N.C.O. and his mate to keep them in order. The roads were in a bad state for we were in the region of the Dortmund–Ems canal. How many times back in England had we heard the news broadcaster announce that the Dortmund–Ems canal had been successfully bombed yet again. We were looking at the result. Railway lines were gathered together in grotesque knots. Fallen telegraph poles looped about with wires lay among the debris like giant knitting needles. It was late afternoon before we arrived in Wettringen through streets that emptied at our approach. The fleeting glimpse of an alarmed face at a window suggested that we had taken the townsfolk by surprise, an impression that was confirmed as we drove through the iron gates of the orphanage which had been requisitioned for our use. Abandoned clothing littered the steps: a ruck-sack, hurriedly packed and then forgotten, a German helmet with a crumpled letter inside, a stretcher upturned over stained blankets.

The confusion was worse inside the building. It had already been used as a hospital by the Germans who had almost been caught napping by the speed of our advance. Their order to pull out had come only that morning, in the middle of breakfast, if the plates of congealed eggs and bacon were anything to judge by. The patients had been hastily plucked from their beds, leaving bedpans unemptied and wash-bowls full of scummy water.

I was given a long basement room containing twenty used beds and a formidable stench, since all the windows were impenetrably sealed with sandbags. We were to be operational by the next morning and it was now five p.m. I took a deep breath and hoped that the host hospital was providing a strong, strapping orderly for me. What I got was a solemn, skinny little 'spelk' with enormous boots who looked as though he could not lift a pillow, never mind the dead weight of an unconscious man.

'Private Bonepart, Sister,' he said, taking off his jacket and tightening his belt. 'Spelt differently.'

He was no bigger than I, and nobody was as small as that. 'Then this could be your Waterloo,' I sighed. I must make the best of it. At least he looked intelligent. We would make up in brains what we lacked in brawn. 'We have to change this into a working ward by tomorrow.'

Things began to happen. Somebody's C.O. sent two Pioneers to help me and I had them take away the filthy, rotting sandbags and prise open the screwed-down windows. We flung open the double doors on the ramp leading to a lawn outside and out went mattresses and pillows for an airing, letting in a sharp breeze that raised goose-pimples and cleared away the smells. 'Boney' produced soap, buckets of hot water and scrubbing brushes and I soon realised what a treasure I had. My little orderly and I worked as one. There was no need for me to instruct for he knew exactly what there was to be done. We stripped the beds of their dirty linen and swept and scrubbed the floors and lockers, set up a treatment table and appropriated extra instruments and a superb dressing trolley from the German operating theatre. Boney was the first to hear that a room full of linen had been discovered and returned from successive forays with arms full of sheets, towels and pillow-slips, each prominently marked with a swastika. Our own War Department supplies were adequate but never generous. These extra items would allow us to be more liberal with sheet changing.

We decided that the raised platform at one end of the room should be our work area and Boney looted a small cupboard from somewhere for our tea and milk supplies. Predictably, he had a friend in the cookhouse who saw us right in this matter. With the addition of a primus stove and a jerrycan of water, we made a kitchen for dispensing hot drinks to the patients (and, incidentally, ourselves) whenever necessary. My office desk was an upturned crate just large enough to hold the Admission and Report Books, temperature charts and requisition forms for diet, dispensary and Quartermaster's stores.

By the time we had made up the beds afresh and sterilised instruments and syringes, the day was almost gone but I could tell Major Fitzgibbon that we were ready to receive patients. Profoundly pleased with ourselves but dead on our feet, we locked the doors to the ward and climbed the steps in search of supper and bed.

'You take the lamp, Boney.' The Engineers were still working on power lines which the departing Germans had cut. 'You have further to walk.' The sisters were quartered in the building itself but the men were under canvas on the nearby Sportzplatz. I handed him the hurricane lamp and wondered if I looked as weary as he did. 'Baby Boney', his mates called him, but it was only a baby face until you noticed the set of his jaw. Now he was heavy-eyed. He took the lamp with a nod.

'See you tomorrow then. Grand opening.'

I went in search of our Mess through dim, unfamiliar passages and I could hear Boney trying to clatter quietly in his big boots as he made for the exit. Eyes at the windows of houses near by would be watching his lantern as he crossed the football field. German people living near the tents would hear English voices in their midst as our men cooked beans and bangers, scrubbed their mess-tins, sluiced themselves under the trees.

I found food left for me in a deserted dining-room, the nursing staff of the general hospital having retired to bed, although my two colleagues in the 'Max-Factor' theatre were still sterilising equipment ready for the next morning.

'Top floor, Sister. Room Number Six.' The Mess orderly handed me a candle. 'You'll find your kit there ready.'

It was said that the orphanage had been a home for carefully bred Aryan boys, the product of unions between Hitler's élite, stormtroopers and selected maidens of pure nordic physical attributes. In a lakeside setting not far away was a spacious maternity home where these super-babies were reputed to have been born. When the Germans made the orphanage into a hospital the children were accommodated by people in the village. We had remarked upon the little blonde boys who had watched our arrival with curiosity from the safety of garden fences in nearby houses.

Now, as I climbed the stairs to a dark and silent passage on the top floor, my flickering candle fell on framed texts and heroic pictures, of German warriors defeating mythical beasts in Wagnerian landscapes, and illuminated verse urging every good boy to fight for the Fatherland.

Most of the doors I passed were closed, their inmates no doubt asleep, but one stood open and tempted my curiosity. It was the school mending room. Inside were sewing machines with torn sheets still under the needle: pins, scissors and tape measures just as the needlewoman had left them. Another room was stacked with small shoes and here, at last, was a bonus for being small. An excellent pair of leather sandals fitted me perfectly and I had no compunction about taking them. It did not seem like stealing.

I found Number Six further along the passage and gingerly turned the handle. Inside, an apprehensive face stared back at me from a ghostly mirror over a chest of drawers, a tired face with untidy hair. I set my candle down amongst pots of face cream left behind by some 'schwester' in her haste to leave. There was a bottle of self-confident perfume and hair pins strong enough to hold a horse's tail. Her huge, billowing, down-filled

bed was just as she had leapt from it. Someone had laid
out a couple of clean sheets for me but I could not face making
even one more bed that night and untied my bedroll instead,
to sleep on the floor.

The casualties came in down the ramp next morning.
Facially injured men were carried either propped upright or
lying face downwards on crooked arm. Lying flat on his back,
a man's tongue would fall back to block his windpipe. This was
another lesson from the First World War. Our new ward
presented easy access for the stretcher bearers. Ambulances
could back right to the door on the ramp then it was only a few
steps to the waiting beds. We kept one side of the ward for pre-
operative resuscitation, and here Boney and I received them
between grey blankets, resuscitated and washed them and
prepared them for the theatre. On their return from the theatre,
the men were lifted into clean sheets on the other side of the
ward, in the recovery position, without pillows, until they
came round from anaesthesia. During this potentially dangerous
time, we had to keep a close watch for heart or respiratory failure and the slight figure of Major Thornton, the anaesthetist,
was a common enough sight, still in theatre gown, concernedly
bent over the inert forms of men newly brought from the
operating table, their rubber airways still in position.

The surgeons helped whenever they were free, heaving helpless men up on their pillows, watching an unconscious man
while I did a round of penicillin injections. Boney was in six
places at once. I was repeatedly late for meals, a fact that sometimes annoyed our host Matron, but it was unavoidable. There
were times when Boney could not be left to cope on his own and
vice versa. I hardly saw the theatre sisters who were as fully
stretched as I was myself. We worked willingly and with fresh
hope now for American and British troops were overrunning the
country and there was news of a powerful Russian drive from
the East. Germany was in a hopeless position.

Towards the latter half of April, casualties in the area began
to tail off and we prepared for another move forward, this time to
Celle in Lower Saxony, about 150 miles away. Before we left,

a few of us were able to spend a day at the newly-opened Rest Centre, the old maternity home, where we met front line troops from the battles of the Rhine and the Elbe, justifiably relaxing. We swam in the lake, played table tennis and danced until the early hours to a German string quartet determinedly showing a brave face to the conquerors. They were better off than most civilians. At least they were given a good meal and the occasional cigarette which was much too valuable to smoke. It would be wrapped carefully in a pocket handkerchief and hidden away in an inside pocket. On the black market, cigarettes already commanded a respectful barter value.

I took my leave of Boney. I think he was as sorry as I that the partnership was breaking up. We had worked together in rare agreement since that first morning nearly three weeks ago. Set apart from the rest of the hospital, we had each depended implicitly on co-operation from the other. Had he been a less able orderly, I could not have run the busy ward with such harmony. Boney was another pair of hands, gentle and patient, never needing a reminder: another pair of ears to pick up the change in a man's breathing, and eyes to detect the beginning of tell-tale blueness from air obstruction. He never absented himself on long, mysterious errands which, for most orderlies, usually ended with an illicit cigarette behind the incinerator, and when I would be nearly dropping with tiredness, Boney would be up there on the platform, busy with the primus. 'Tea break, Sister.' In peacetime, Mr. Bonepart was a school teacher with an aversion to war. In wartime, he was a first-class nurse.

Celle was a large town with wide streets which had got off lightly in the bombing raids. Its gas training centre set in pleasant grounds offered ample accommodation for a 600-bed hospital. On 25th April, the 121st B.G.H. moved into 'Heergaschenschule' and the Maxillo-Facial unit, still in conjunction with the 'Heads' unit, moved in the same day.

Here were large, airy classrooms which would adapt easily into wards and, for us, the comfortable sleeping quarters of trainee German officers. But we fell silent when we came to the basement of our new location which had been, until recently, the

scene of research into that dreaded dimension of warfare–
gas. Flasks and phials and huge Jeroboams full of evil-looking
fluids winked and glimmered in a succession of laboratories.
The protective clothing department was like some ghoulish
fancy-dress wardrobe: rubber suits with fish-like fins, head-
pieces with obscene snouts and row upon row of giant thigh
boots. Before we opened as a hospital, all these macabre
reminders were removed.

For a ward, I was given a classroom with sink and running
water, a blackboard and a Bunsen burner, a great improvement on my last accommodation. Before going in search of my
new Matron, I climbed on a chair and wiped the blackboard clean of chemical equations and formulae. In their place
I wrote, Maxillo-Facial Ward 1945.

There were two letters awaiting me at Celle, one from Pin
who was still with the 108th in Brussels but expecting to move
up into Germany in the near future. She sent news of our
friends in the 75th. Duff, Annie P. Scott, Joan Deadman and
Margaret Fairy had all been posted to India and more postings
were anticipated now that operations in Europe were tailing off.
The war against Japan showed no signs of ending and South-
East Asia Command was increasing the number of hospitals in
India to accommodate casualties air-lifted from Burma. The
other letter dealt with the same subject. It was from Pat Fuller.
We had corresponded regularly ever since I left Brussels and
had managed one brief assignment on the airfield at Eindhoven by
courtesy of the pilot who flew the Forces' mail. His previous letters
had spoken of his possible posting to South-East Asia Command
and this one confirmed it. He was leaving Brussels immediately
on embarkation leave in England before sailing to India.

'You'll be out there soon,' he assured me. 'Europe's finished.
Do your best to get on the draft for India.'

But my job with the 'Max-Factors' was by no means finished.
My classroom ward quickly filled with a different category of
patients. Hordes of joyful British prisoners of war were being
released every day as German camps and hospitals were over-
run. Among them were Maxillo-Facial cases whose initial

surgery had been carried out by German doctors. They were dirty and hungry when they came to us, their bandages filthy and many of the wounds septic but all were in such excellent spirits at finding themselves once more in British hands that they made light of their sufferings. The surgery, in most cases, had been conscientiously carried out, but lack of drugs, and especially penicillin, had resulted in foul, suppurating wounds. Pat Kavanagh, a tall, fair Irish sister from the 121st was sent to help me with the time-consuming dressings and together we made a start.

We began with penicillin injections all round, then antiseptic mouthwashes for their white-coated tongues and hot saline packs on their septic wounds. Many would have to go back to the theatre to have abscesses drained and maladjusted jaws placed under traction but nothing could spoil the contentment of their first night of freedom. Our Catering Officer did the right thing and sent up a crate of captured champagne so that each man could celebrate his release, even if it meant slobbering through a straw wedged in splinted jaws. Only the chap with the nasal tube looked put out. He found no elation whatever in the draught we poured down his funnel, only wind.

Understandably enough, we were thoroughly hated by the inhabitants of Celle. When we went into the town, accompanied by the obligatory armed guard, civilians pointedly crossed to the other side of the street and the glances that came our way were openly hostile.

A shocking rumour sprang up in the hospital, so horrible it could not be believed. Then some of our doctors were asked to go to a nearby place called Belsen where a concentration camp had been discovered containing such unimaginable horrors that soldiers hardened to war's worst sights were sickened. Medical units moved in to salvage what they could but deliverance came too late for the thousands of men, women and children who had already perished in the gas chamber.

Our M.O.s came back with photographs so we knew it was all true. The Nazi guards, some of them women, had been ordered to bury the dead. We saw a photograph of them slinging emaciated corpses into a deep pit already half-filled. Their faces registered no horror at the task. British army units set about clearing up the camp and helping the dazed and sick survivors, some of whom found their way to Celle.

Pat Kavanagh and I were returning from an escorted walk when we saw these grotesque creatures for the first time. Dressed in striped cotton jacket and trousers, the unmistakable camp uniform, they wandered aimlessly at the edge of the town, poking about in drains and refuse bins. Their stick-like limbs seemed scarcely able to support swollen, drum-tight bellies. Their eyes were nothing more than deep-set sockets in a shaven skull from which all flesh had long since shrunk. They leaned over railings, and stared in at the windows of houses. Pat and I were horrified. The inhabitants of Celle drew away as if from lepers, preferring not to acknowledge this disgusting evidence of crimes committed no further than ten miles from their doorsteps. Their indifference was so marked that a documentary film of the camp was shown in the town with compulsory attendance for every adult German.

They were queueing outside the cinema under the eye of a British Military Policeman as Pat and I passed by.

'They don't look too upset,' she remarked.

For the old folk in the queue, it was just one more hideous disillusionment with a régime which they had followed like sheep. Possibly they would not believe what they were about to see and were too involved with their own suffering to care. Some of the young people there had faces moulded by Hitler, cruel, scornful and overbearing, and they smirked with bravado behind the M.P.'s back.

The end was near. On 30th April, Hitler committed suicide and all German units capitulated immediately. The last guns left a loaded silence, their waiting crews not yet able to believe that the fighting was really over. There was to be a radio broadcast to the nation and all the Forces by the Prime Minister, Winston Churchill. A loudspeaker was rigged up by the swimming pool in the 'gas school' grounds. Ward radios were tuned in, and as the moment approached, not a sound was heard, not a patient asked for a drink or a bottle. There was a deep, expectant hush and a lump in the throat of each of us as the familiar voice began to speak, no longer steeling us for yet more privations nor thundering dire threats against the Nazis. The voice that had injected into the nation the strength to defy Hitler was touched now with deep emotion as he told us all what we desperately wanted to hear. After six long years of hardship and misery, the war with Germany was over.

In the ward, our poor botched-up, patched-up ex-P.O.W.s hurrayed as well as they could through clamped jaws and the whole hospital joined in the singing of the National Anthem. The German cleaners looked sourly away.

The war had ended. We kept reminding ourselves. No more killing and maiming and mutilating. The war in Europe was over.

After the rejoicing came the reckoning. War had cut a swathe of devastation across Europe leaving huge problems for the victors to solve. The homeless must be housed, the sick cared for and the dead must be given a proper burial. The Allied War Graves Commission set about their task of identifying the dead and constructing suitable cemeteries. They did not overlook the corner of a field in Hermanville near the site of the F.D.S. Today there is a memorial there to all the men we could not save. Sheltering cypresses have grown up to make it a green corner of remembrance.

The International Red Cross began the work, that has lasted to the present day, of reuniting broken families. The refugees from Hitler's armament factories, mines and oil refineries from places as far apart as Poland and France, Lithuania and Bavaria, Czechoslovakia and Belgium, his subjugated labour force, were now adrift on a chaotic continent. Their homes were gone, the whereabouts of their families unknown. Euphemistically referred to as 'Displaced Persons', they were given food and shelter in temporary camps run by the Allied armies and the Red Cross. But the D.P. camp became home for thousands of people. The young met and married there and eventually took a gamble together when a new life was offered in Australia or

Canada. They put their past behind them. Many never saw their families again nor knew whether they were alive or not. Even today, the International Red Cross, working laboriously through mountains of official documents, can sometimes bring about the miraculous reunion between an old man and his Australian grandson, an old woman and her young Canadian descendants.

The survivors of the concentration camps presented a more difficult problem. Rehabilitation into a free world was going to be a slow process and any improvement in their physical condition would not be brought about easily. Many were already close to death and their reprieve was only temporary.

For us who, at that time, were not closely involved with the tragedy of the concentration camps, life at the 121st B.G.H. became much more relaxed. On V.E. night, 8th May, there was a bonfire party with fireworks in the hospital grounds and high jinks at midnight in the swimming pool, but even after V.E. day, the holiday mood persisted. There were no more long convoys of ambulances with their swinging 'Casualty' boards. New cases came in singly now and were usually the result of traffic accidents or carelessness with weapons. We had more time to spend on the men already in the wards and grafting was begun on burns and other injuries where skin cover was urgent.

At the beginning of June, we held a hospital swimming regatta and several interesting facts emerged about people we thought we knew so well. One of our dental mechanics was an expert at the crawl, while Sister Bell and Major Holland were assets to anybody's team, ploughing up the water like dreadnoughts. Major Fitzgibbon did not like water and would not take his clothes off. Tommy Gibson could not swim for toffee. It was a period of welcome relaxation for us. Life was easy through the long summer days. Our off-duty time was pleasantly passed with the occasional picnic or visit to neighbouring army messes. Tommy Gibson, with time on his hands in the theatre one day, said the scar on my neck from a gland excision when I was a child, was a disgrace to a plastic surgery unit and promptly cut it out under a local anaesthetic. Olivia Holmes and Vaughan-Jones hastened to conceal any little defect either of them might happen to have as Tommy's eye looked around for further practice.

But we could not go on like this. There was still a war in South-East Asia where men's faces were being injured and in the first week of June, the 'Max-Factors' were recalled to England, to re-equip for India. But I was not to go with them. This time a ward sister was not allowed for and I had to wave them goodbye. With them went my chance of joining Pat Fuller.

'At least you've got a better neck than when we found you,' said Tommy Gibson as the trucks bore the Maxillo-Facial unit away.

Almost immediately, Pat Kavanagh and myself were posted to join the 86th B.G.H. at Rotenburg, a small town some thirty miles east of Bremen, and this posting was to be unlike any other we had known. We were to nurse men just released from Sandbostel, a concentration camp in the north of Germany.

14

After the Concentration Camps: Rotenburg

We drove through the main street of Celle for the last time, Pat
Kavanagh and I and the driver, in a Utility truck bound for
Rotenburg, a distance of about fifty miles. Our road took us
through the chaos that had become commonplace, wrecked
railways, burnt-out trams, ruined houses. Weary civilians
sorted through heaps of rubble in search of re-usable building
material. Their plight was wretched. They were short of food
and the mark as currency was a useless piece of paper. Only
cigarettes or penicillin had purchasing power.

A German cleaner in the hospital at Celle had landed herself
in great trouble by saving cigarette ends from patients' ashtrays
with the intention of recovering the unsmoked tobacco and
selling it. Smoke seeping from under the cupboard where her
cleaning materials were kept gave the game away. Her smould-
ering hoard was discovered in the subsequent fire alert and she
lost her precious job.

Leaving the low-lying valley of the River Weser behind, we
came to high, lightly wooded healthlands and here, near the
town of Rotenburg, we found our new unit, a settlement of
single storey timber buildings amongst pine trees and low gorse
scrub. This had been a German Red Cross centre for convalescent soldiers. Now its function was to provide shelter for
victims of the concentration camps. It was a place of peace and
tranquillity. Deer cropped the bracken at the edge of the woods
and there were rabbits and hares on the sandy heath. Pleasantly
surprised with the location, Pat and I went in search of the
Matron of our new hospital to report our arrival.

'Can't wait to see the wards,' said Pat, looking towards the
long, wooden buildings.

Our new Matron was younger than the average and made
the rules very elastic in order to compensate for the joylessness

of our work. 'Tomorrow will be soon enough,' she said. 'Come and have a drink with me before dinner.'

There was a small staff of sisters and a comfortable Mess. Pat and I shared a twin-bedded room that looked out to the edge of a wood noisy with wood-pigeons. It might have been the first day of a summer holiday in the country.

The next day, dressed in grey cotton frocks, head veils lifting in the breeze, we reported to our respective wards to meet our new patients. Some were in bed, some lay sprawled on top of the beds and others wandered idly about the compound. These men no longer wore the infamous striped clothes of the camp and had been issued with Red Cross pyjamas, but in other respects, they were indistinguishable from the poor wrecks we had seen in Celle. They had the same hollow eyes, shaven skulls, limbs without flesh, the same distended abdomens. Bowed and emaciated, they were hardly recognisable as civilised men, yet I was to learn later that amongst them were musicians and doctors, writers and philosophers, now because of their political beliefs or an accident of birth reduced by man's inhumanity to the level of survivors.

Sister Davies was the tall, attractive sister in charge of the ward where I was to work. In answer to my question about the diagnoses of these men she threw up her hands.

'Each one is a walking textbook. Most of them have heart complications and kidney failure. Some of them are tubercular. They're all anaemic and they've all got sores. We plug along as well as we can.'

I tried to make some contact with these silent and withdrawn men as I pushed my dressing trolley to their beds, but their faces were full of mistrust, and cunning with fear. They dropped their eyes in front of my smile and pushed away the hand I stretched out to help. Their release from horror was still too new. They were in a state of shock and had only one instinct left, to survive.

'We don't insist that they stay in bed,' said Sister Davies when I could not find the owner of a badly ulcerated leg. 'The main thing is for them to feel free.'

So the men with chronic heart disease, bronchitis, stomach ulcers, liver abscesses got up and walked about if they wanted to. They had learned in the camp that the man who is too ill to get up and work soon found himself in the gas chamber and the habit was hard to break. They still had not fully grasped that their Nazi jailors were gone forever.

This was certainly nursing with a difference and it brought very few rewards. Ulcers and sores would not readily heal on men so reduced in health and strength. Temperatures stayed up and so did blood pressures. Haemoglobin levels in the blood stayed dangerously low but, as Sister Davies had said, there was nothing else to do but plug on.

It seemed to me that anything we might do would be a drop in the ocean but we determinedly pressed on with treatments. We handed out vitamin tablets and cough mixtures, urinary antiseptics and iron pills. I dressed their sores each day but all I got back was indifference. There was not the slightest exchange of human feeling between us those first days. It was hard going.

'It'll get better,' said the M.O. This was his second camp.

We were nursing Lithuanians, Poles, German Jews and one solitary Frenchman. We had to pick up the common tongue, a sort of bastard German, in order to communicate. Even then, we never really knew whether we had been understood or not. The dead eyes rarely kindled with a response.

The one exception was a German named Kaiser. Strangely, this man never stopped talking to anyone who would listen. He was a rat-faced little man with a mouthful of gold teeth which, in itself, was highly suspicious. In the camps, no-one was left with gold in his head unless he was on good terms, very good terms, with his Nazi jailors. The things he told us were horrible. The prisoners had been forced to swallow a large dose of castor oil each day which weakened still further their debilitated condition and at the same time provided sport for the guards who enjoyed shooting at the pale targets squatting over the latrine trenches. I believed what he told me.

Kaiser was one of the few patients who could speak English, and rejoiced in the status of interpreter. I found it hard to feel pity for this man. He fawned for favours in a way that made my flesh creep. His ingratiating antics made me feel sick, and it was was noticeable that his fellow prisoners gave him a wide berth. I could carry out all manner of attentions on the gruesome bodies of the others but I could not help recoiling from contact with the scabby flesh of this gabbling monkey-man with his flashing gold teeth and impertinent eyes.

There was one man who never left his bed. This was the Frenchman who had lost a leg in the camp and was in a very poor way. He lay, propped on his pillows all day, pale as a lily, drained by successive haemorrhages, with only the faintest flicker of awareness in his light grey eyes. Even they seemed to have had the colour washed from them.

Although the patients had the freedom to wander at will within the compound of the hospital, they were always back in the ward at mealtimes, no matter where they had strayed, silently converging on the food trolley with their tin plates, eyes rivetted on the containers full of meat and vegetables. The helpings had to be small at first for their shrunken stomachs could not take normal rations. Despite the regular meals, Sister Davies and I would find, while making the beds, a slice of corned beef, a potato or a piece of bread hidden under a pillow, for they could not yet be sure that another day would bring more food.

Sometimes we despaired for these men. What future was there for them? No-one knew where their families were and they themselves seemed to have forgotten that they ever had wives or children. They only cared for the food trolley. Every other instinct or emotion had been suppressed except the will to survive.

Pat and I discussed the problem in the evenings after duty as we sat in the recreation room looking out on the peaceful summer landscape.

'If only they'd understand that we're trying to help them.'

'Our M.O. says that will come. Got to give them time.'

German medical orderlies were drafted to help us, as a form of retribution, but I could hardly bear to work with them, and when they proved themselves more efficient than our homely British orderlies, who were beginning to think of demobilisation, I disliked them more than ever. The morning cup of coffee brought by our British orderly was a not-too-clean cup on a sloppy saucer, but the German orderly improvised a tray and cut a doyley from a piece of foolscap.

'Greasing to the sister,' grumbled our man audibly and scuffed off to get his tea from the cookhouse.

Then my hard line towards Germans was upset by the arrival of the German Red Cross nurses. A civilian van arrived in the compound one day and a cheerful bunch of young girls wearing Red Cross armbands jumped down. They lived in Bremen and had volunteered to help nurse the camp victims. I remembered the giggling adolescents in the cinema queue at Celle, and did not return the engaging smile of seventeen-year-old Rosa when the Sergeant Major brought her over.

Feeling hard as nails, I marched her off and spared her nothing, the matchstick legs and broken bodies indelibly stamped with the camp number. I showed her the Frenchman who had been left lying around at the camp after a botched-up amputation and who now had a sore on his backside big enough to put a fist in. Transparent with anaemia, he sat plucking the bedclothes with waxy fingers. The young girl looked in horror and began to cry, and my face flooded with guilt. I was behaving no better than the Nazis.

'You can help me bath him,' I said, more kindly, 'and I'll show you how to dress his bedsore.'

'We didn't know,' said Rosa, dropping warm tears on the hand of the wondering Frenchman. 'As God is my witness, in Bremen we did not know.'

The Red Cross girls came every day in their puffing-billy truck and worked until they dropped with tiredness, getting small thanks and expecting none.

Sunshine and fresh air, careful diet and medical attention at last began to bring about encouraging signs of improvement. Ulcers, static for weeks, began to grow in from the edges with healthy, pink granulations. Bronchitis and dysentery were brought under control. Hair thickened on shaven heads and stringy muscles toughened. There was a new spirit in the ward, something very like cheerfulness. The men talked amongst themselves now, and, although they did not actually address us, they no longer looked on us with suspicion. Their eyes showed interest in their surroundings and Davies and I would find them covertly watching us as we went about the ward. Sometimes we overheard ourselves being discussed and it was, quite naturally, 'Grosse Schwester' and 'Kleine Schwester'. They surprised the M.O. one day when he came looking for us on the ward. While I was away taking a coffee break, Davies had cut her finger rather badly on a glass ampoule and so had hurried to the Casualty room to have it stitched.

'Wo ist die Schwester?' the M.O. asked, and a Pole, playing cards with his countrymen, who had obviously missed none of the drama, volunteered with a smile:

'Kleine Schwester Kaffee trinken,

Grosse Schwester kranke Fingern.'

It was an indication of the friendly co-operation that was increasing every day.

My particular problem was a Lithuanian who rejected help at every turn. He had a badly ulcerated leg which needed rest and frequent dressings, but whenever I arrived with the dressing trolley, he was nowhere to be found, and when I pleaded with him to rest his leg a little more, he responded by limping away into the compound. He hated me to touch his leg or any part of him, and it worried me that I could not get his trust. He was always roaming in the trees in his Canadian Red Cross slippers and pyjamas, the most solitary of all these solitary men, and I wondered who he had been before the camp claimed him. At one time, he must have been a tall, well-built man but now his spare frame was bent and humped. Set deep beneath a high forehead, his eyes were as revealing as bits of blue slate. He was a disturbing man and I was a little afraid of him.

One day, I had to face him quite alone when he had wandered a little way from the ward. I could have called an orderly, of course, but that would not have been very good for the relationship that I was trying to build up.

As usual, he had absented himself at the time for his leg dressing and I left my trolley by his bedside to go in search of him. I found him under a pine tree examining the corky bark as if he had never seen a tree before. He hadn't heard my approach and I spoke quietly so as not to alarm him. 'Selzinski, I want to dress your leg.'

He turned abruptly at the sound of my voice and his face coloured with anger. I had intruded into a very private moment and he would not forgive me for that, but I had other patients who needed treatment and I hoped that he would come along quietly. I saw his jugular vein swell up and the thought crossed my mind that he would give himself a coronary if he did not calm down. He shuffled towards me with his neck stuck out exactly like an advancing tortoise and my heart, too, began to thump a bit.

'Come on,' I said, very much the Sister. 'Stop mucking about. I have other men to see to besides yourself,' and I started to walk back to the ward, hoping that he would follow. He did, of course. He got the message even though he probably had not understood the words. The steam went out of him and he limped back to the ward in his customary attitude of hopelessness.

'You two been for a walk?' Davies looked up from the Pathology forms she was indexing.

'Not exactly,' I said tersely. I regretted the incident. It built another barrier between us and I was sorry to have intruded. One had to be a psychiatrist as well as a nurse when dealing with men like these.

The only man in the ward ever to receive a visitor was the Frenchman. A dapper, red-haired major from the French army came one day and sat beside his countryman, clearly upset by his deplorable condition, for here, without a doubt, was a man who could not recover, in spite of all we could do for him. The Major came back a day later with a punnet of strawberries, but the sick man could make no gesture beyond a wan smile. Like a devoted mother with an ailing child, the bristly Major squashed the strawberries on a plate and patiently fed him from a spoon.

'C'est bon, n'est-ce pas?' he crooned. Tenderly he mopped up with his own spotless handkerchief the red stain on the sick man's trembling lip.

A few days later, the Frenchman died. There had never been any hope of saving him. There was no real reason for the ginger Major to come back, but I found him hanging around the Sisters' Mess one day, waiting to intercept me as I went to lunch. He had a splendid suggestion for my next day off. He would take me for a picnic in the countryside. I jumped at the chance. It was not easy for us to get away from the hospital. Pat and I had been to Hamburg once where we had a memorable, but not to be repeated, meeting with some very uninhibited Russians in the Officers' Club. Besides, Hamburg was a burnt-out, depressing place and we had seen enough bomb damage, so the chance of a picnic in the country, away from patients and the ruins of war, was immensely appealing to me.

He drove up a week later, smart as paint in a requisitioned Mercedes. Pat pulled a face at me. 'Doesn't look your type.'

It was a beautiful day in high summer and we drove out of the forested area to farmlands with grazing cattle and ripening corn. My escort spread a rug and as I watched him fussily wedging a bottle of wine to cool in a running stream, I reflected on my luck in finding a Frenchman to take me on a picnic. He had provided fresh bread rolls and a dish of pâté, a cooked chicken wrapped in a napkin with sprigs of tarragon and lovage, and soft, bloomy peaches. An Englishman, with his usual lack of imagination, would have said, 'You bring the eats. I'll bring the booze.'

I took off my jacket and let the sun soak through my silk shirt. With a chicken leg in one hand and a glass of Liebfraumilch in the other. I could find nothing wrong with the world. My garlicky Major tickled my ear with his whiskers. 'Ma chèrie, you like this peeque-neeque?'

The lazy afternoon slid into a golden evening and it was time to pack up and return to the hospital, but when we walked back to the lane where we had parked the car, we found all four wheels firmly sunk in the soft ground.

With annoyance stamped all over his face, the Major put the car into gear and accelerated. The wheels spun round throwing out great gobs of earth but the car sank deeper and deeper.

'Push!' he yelled at me and I pushed. He revved. The deeper the car sank, the crosser he became. But my carefree mood of the afternoon was not to be dispelled so easily. I sank back on the grass, helpless with laughter. This made my friend very terse indeed. Finally, he climbed out of the car, slammed the door and set off to walk to a nearby farm for help. There was nothing I could do, so I stretched out on the grass again to await his return and ponder on how I was to get back to the hospital if the car refused to budge.

He came back a little while later driving before him a horse and two frightened old people. He had found them at a farm and demanded their assistance. My gallant companion of the afternoon was transformed. As if directing an army, he shouted at the old farmer to fasten the horse to the front bumper of the Mercedes. The woman was told to lead it by the bridle while the old man pushed from behind. They strained and pulled, the woman tearful now, tugging the floundering horse. The Major grabbed the whip from the woman's hands and brought it down again and again on the horse's quivering flanks, narrowly missing the old woman. The old man wheezed and gasped. The horse whinnied with fright. It was like some bizarre Italian opera. Outraged, I glared at the Major, unable to believe this could be my charming companion of the 'peeque-neeque'. At last, with a squelching heave, the wheels were pulled free and the car moved on to firm ground.

The Major climbed inside. 'Move your horse or I'll run it over.' The old couple stumbled to untie the rope.

I went to fetch the picnic basket and looked across at them as they stood trembling with fright. 'Danke schön,' I nodded towards them and climbed into the car.

'There's no need to thank them,' the Major said testily. 'You

British are soft in the head.' Needless to say, I never saw my Gallic Romeo again.

By the end of July, the condition of some patients had improved sufficiently for them to be transferred to a Displaced Persons' Camp as the next step in rehabilitation. Here their background would be investigated and every effort made to re-unite them with their families. Those on the transfer list, how-ever, were thrown into utter dejection at the news.

'Soon you will be going home,' we tried to explain, but 'home' was a word they had forgotten. Home was here, in this familiar ward with us. At last they had learned to trust us. We were the only family they wanted to know about and they did not want to leave.

The orderly gave each man a pair of good boots and thick socks. 'Try these for size. Strip your beds. You're moving on.' But the boots and the socks stayed where they were, on the floor.

Selzinski, my troublesome patient, seemed especially affected. He had made a considerable recovery and was growing stronger day by day. The ulcer on his leg was almost healed and his temperature chart had shown a steady course for some time now. We had developed a good relationship over the last weeks and all his old antagonism had disappeared. He had appointed himself unpaid, acting, auxiliary orderly, helping to make beds, collect dirty dishes and clean up my dressing trolley after use. He was still very silent and aloof but seemed perfectly content to go on living each day in this way. He took a pride in his appear-ance now, being always properly shaved and he kept his bed, the only place he could call his own, scrupulously neat and tidy. The thought of having to leave it shocked him.

When I went to put a final dressing on his leg, I found him lying with closed eyes on his bed. He had made no move to prepare himself for the transport which would be here within the hour, and his boots lay where the orderly had left them. He looked up as I edged the trolley nearer and I saw something of the old mistrust in his eyes again. I wondered if he fully understood what was going on and tried to explain again, in my pidgin German, that this was to be one step nearer home.

He sat up with a set face and bared his leg. I had no means of knowing whether or not he had understood. I swabbed the old wound and applied clean gauze and strapping.

'It's nearly better.' I looked up and encountered a desperate look.

The orderly came clattering into the ward. 'Will you put your flippin' boots on! The truck'll be here in a minute. What's the matter with you lot?'

Kaiser flashed his golden smile. 'They think it is a trick. In the camp, guards give special clothes, tell people they are seeing wives and sweethearts soon. Only place they go is the gas chamber. Big joke when special clothes come off again.' He threw back his head and laughed and I wondered again about those teeth.

In the end, we had to send for the M.O., and when they saw he meant business, the men who were on the transfer list, which included all Lithuanians, sullenly began to dress. They put on socks and boots and a greatcoat over their pyjamas. All they possessed in the world went into their little cotton Dorothy Bags: a piece of soap maybe, an inch of candle, a comb, a razor and perhaps a pencil. In silence, the remaining patients watched them go slowly out of the ward door.

Sister Davies and I had arranged a little farewell gift for each man. We had scrounged, one way and another, enough cigarettes, chocolate and biscuits to make up a small parcel, including a laboriously compounded message in German. They were received in silence. None of the men batted an eyelid or said a word as, clutching their unopened parcels, they climbed aboard the truck and took their places on the benches inside. It was a sad sort of leavetaking. They believed that we had let them down. The truck's engine throbbed into life and I saw that Selzniksi alone was opening his parcel. Carefully he extracted the note we had enclosed and spread it on his knee.

'God bless you and bring you happiness,' was the message we had tried to convey, and when he looked up he was actually smiling, a crack of a smile. As the truck began to move, he staggered to his feet, clutching at the overhead strut for support.

'Wiedersehen —' he called out in his uncouth, dry voice. 'Wiedersehen und vielen Dank!'

As we happily waved them off, we firmly believed that they were going home, perhaps not straight away, but eventually.

Only later did we realise that Lithuania had ceased to exist as a country, and now the fate of Selzinski and his fellow countrymen leaves me with a question mark.

15

The Return Home

By the beginning of August the last camp victims had gone. The wards were thoroughly cleaned and disinfected before convalescent British soldiers arrived. It was good to hear patients whistling happily and gossiping again after the taciturn men from the camp. A German car was given to the Sisters' Mess for our own use and since I was the only sister with a driving licence, I was in a favoured position to explore the area.

My first expedition was to see Pin. Her last letter had come from Munster, about thirty miles away, where she was nursing orthopaedic cases. It was still forbidden for women to venture abroad without an armed escort so I informed the guard detachment of my proposed trip to Munster and asked for a volunteer to accompany me. To the loud cheers of his mates at the Guardroom window, the private who was 'volunteered' for this task climbed into the back of the Opel and I drove off, somewhat diffidently, I must admit, since I had not driven a car for at least eight years and that had been over the traffic-free moors of Northumberland. German civilians and old ladies on bicycles gave us a wide berth but we reached Pin's mess without mishap. She poked her head into the back of the car. 'Aren't you nervous?' she asked my guard, rather tactlessly, I thought.

'Not at all,' he said agreeably. 'Once we got on to the right side of the road, it was OK.'

I never got the same guard twice on these expeditions.

Six months had gone by since I left Pin in Brussels. The pavements outside the Hotel Regina had been slushy with snow the day I drove away and now it was dusty August in northern Germany. There was a great deal of news to be exchanged. Duff had written to me from Quetta in northern India. She was to be bridesmaid to Margaret Fairy in the near future. Soutie, Pin told me, was in Germany at the steel town of Solingen but her hospital was on the point of departure for India. Until that came about, she was busy fitting out her bottom drawer with a comprehensive range of cutlery.

Military hospitals all over Germany were moving out to India. Only those necessary for the welfare of the occupation troops were to remain and Pin and I knew that it could not be long before we, too, were given embarkation leave.

'And what about your kind man?' Pin asked.

'In India,' I said. 'He's a major now.'

Pin's hospital received orders to pack up a few days after my visit and the 86th was scheduled to follow as soon as the settlement at Rotenburg could be handed back to the German Red Cross. Our convalescent soldiers changed out of their hideous blue 'sick' suits (these, though very patriotic with white shirt and red tie, lacked any dignity whatsoever) and we sent them home for a spell of leave.

One last engagement before we left was an unexpected invitation to dine at the Staff H.Q. of Lt. General Horrocks who was in command of the rehabilitation of this section of Germany. Six of us who were off duty, which included Pat and myself, were collected by the General's staff car and conveyed to the pleasant house which was his H.Q., where musicians waited to play for us and a candelit table was laid for dinner. The General, whose name I had heard spoken with affection and admiration by the soldiers I had nursed from Normandy to Germany, welcomed us with courtesy and charm, and, like the soldiers before me, I became an instant admirer. After the work with concentration camp victims, this happy and civilised evening did much to restore the balance of living.

The dropping of atomic bombs on Japan changed the whole course of the war in the Far East and South-East Asia, and, on 14th August, Japan surrendered. The war was over now throughout the world. But plans for our hospital were not affected. We were still to go to India. A train took us from Bremen slowly and with many stops over recently repaired track to Belgium, to a transit unit in Bruges where we were to

await sailing orders. While we were there, a letter from Pat
Fuller in India threw me into confusion.

'Lucky you never did get out to India,' he wrote. 'My
demob. number is twenty. I should be home for Christmas.'

Gradual demobilisation on the basis of 'first in-first out' had
been going on since the end of the European war. Pat, as a
Territorial, had been called up at the outbreak of hostilities in
1939 and consequently fell into a high priority demobilisation
category. My group number was fifty-two. If I sailed to India,
our ships would probably pass in the Indian Ocean and we
would be unlikely to meet again. I took a long look at our
relationship. What did it amount to anyway? A month spent
jazzing it up in Brussels and a ruck-sack full of letters. It was not
enough to matter, but too much to discard. I went to ask my
C.O., Colonel Lassen, for a posting on compassionate grounds
but he said my case was altogether too flimsy to get me off the
India draft. Dame Louisa Wilkinson, the Chief Queen Bee of all
the Q.A.s, was visiting the area at the time. 'Put your case to
her,' Colonel Lassen advised, 'and wrap it up a bit.'

Dame Louisa had dealt with many Q.A.s in her time. 'I don't
see you wearing a ring,' she said.

I was kept in suspense until the last moment when my reprieve was delivered to the docks at Ostend. The ship carrying
Pat Kavanagh and the rest of the 86th sailed for England leaving me waving farewell on the quay. I reported to a transit
hotel nearby until the War Office should decide what to do with
me.

I had no ring, Dame Louisa was right. I was not even sure
that I wanted one, but I wanted the chance to find out.

Q.A.s on the way to and from postings stopped-over in the
Ostend transit hotel. Most were newly recruited and I was
among the few wearing the old grey and scarlet. One night I
saw a familiar face among the new arrivals, an older woman,
last seen in the long full skirts and starched bonnet of a Sister
Tutor at the Newcastle hospital, looking strangely undressed
now in a short, khaki skirt. Her face showed relief at the sight
of me. The transition from her own place of absolute authority

in the classroom to a number in the army must have been a
difficult one for her. I was not much help. Pettily, I remembered
how she had sent me coughing from the lecture room during my
first few wretched days as a nurse.

Notice of two weeks' leave in England arrived for me. I was
to present myself at 1800 hrs, 28thAugust, to the purser of an
L.S.T. sailing that night from Ostend. This was my second
spell of leave. The first had been in January and we had travel-
led by air, in great comfort compared with the conditions
aboard the L.S.T. I found her full of troops going on leave, a
handful of officers and three other Q.A.s apart from myself.
We four were shown along a narrow catwalk in the deep interior of the vessel to bunks on the side of a great hold packed with
troops. It was hard to believe that this was where we were
expected to sleep. There was no light, no air, no privacy, and
my stomach turned over in anticipation of the ship's motion
down here. It was to be the *Invicta* all over again.

The purser was harassed and not very interested in our complaints. His deck cabins, he said, were already allocated, to
senior officers, we presumed, and he pointed out that we did
have a curtain to screen off our sleeping recess. I burned with
indignation. There were no other women in the hold. Nothing
could have persuaded me to sleep there knowing as I did that I
would be laid out with seasickness after the first five minutes.
But my three colleagues seemed resigned to their fate and took
to their bunks as the ship left port. I made my way up on deck,
intending to spend the night there.

As soon as we were out into the Channel, the ship began to
roll. It was not a particularly rough sea and a conventional
vessel would have ridden smoothly over the waves, but the flat
bottom of the L.S.T. produced a curious wallowing motion
which filled me with a dreadful presentiment. I gripped the rail
tightly and swallowed hard, trying not to think what it must be
like down below.

It was dark now but fortunately, since I was to spend the
night out here, not cold. Apart from members of the crew going
about their business, the deck was deserted. I watched the dark

waves as they dipped and swelled and thought longingly of a horizontal bunk.

A voice over the ship's loudspeaker startled me. 'Will a nursing sister please report to the Sick Bay immediately. This is urgent. Repeat. This is urgent.'

I did not want to believe what I heard. I was not in a fit condition to look after anyone. Quite the reverse. I felt aggrievedly that someone should be looking after me. Going below to consult the other three Q.A.s, I found them looking bleary-eyed over the basins they held.

'I wondered which one of us . . .' I began, but it was useless to pretend. They were pea-green and understandably unconcerned about the rest of the passengers. Down here in the hold, the ship's motion was devilish as she lifted and smacked down her flat bottom on every rising wave. I hurried away to find the Sick Bay.

It was a small cubbyhole in the bowels of the ship. There were two bunks and a tray of clinical instruments, a splint or two and a cupboard labelled POISON. A naval rating with Sick Berth Attendant spelt out on his armband was standing at the side of a man who lay groaning on one of the bunks.

'Is there no doctor on board?' I asked the deck officer who brought me down. But of course there wasn't, or a sister would not have been requested. 'What's the history, then?'

The man had complained of pain shortly after sailing and it had got steadily worse. I turned his unbuttoned trousers down and removed the hands clutching his abdomen. There, on the right side, was a scar. That was my first bit of luck.

'When did you have your appendix out?'

'Last year, Sister.' That was one possible emergency ruled out.

I became aware of an alteration in the rhythm of the ship's engines. We had changed to Slow Ahead. Suddenly a ferocious looking man with a lot of gold stripes on his arm was standing behind me. My deck officer came to a smart salute and I was introduced to the Captain of the ship. He informed me coldly that the leave of all troops on board was in my hands. We were not yet halfway across the Channel. How ill was the man? Should the ship go about and return him to hospital in Ostend? Or take a chance and continue?

I turned back to the man, trying not to be influenced by the enormity of my decision. I felt his head, took his pulse. He was in great discomfort but not, I thought, excruciating pain. The site of the pain could mean a ruptured ulcer but there was no typical rigidity of the abdomen. Suddenly I caught a whiff of his breath and bent down closer to his face.

'Which were you last night?'

He opened one bloodshot eye and winked. 'Father and Mother of a party, Sister.'

'What were you drinking?'

'Belgian plonk,' and he groaned afresh, clutching at his middle.

I turned to the Captain. 'There'll be no need to turn back. You can continue,' I said grandly. It was not a bit of use his trying to overawe me. I did not like his manner and I did not like the type of courtesy shown to Q.A.s on his ship.

'You'd better be sure,' he said, with a touch of a threat in his voice.

'I am,' I said. 'He's suffering from alcoholic poisoning.' I turned once more to my patient.

The sick berth attendant brought me a basin and I instructed the patient to thrust two fingers down his throat. At once I had to share the basin with him. The Sick Bay was somewhere near the screw and the movement down there was worse than anything I could have imagined. The Captain and his entourage beat a hasty retreat and I never saw him again.

'Poor Sister,' my patient squinted at me through running eyes. 'You didn't even have a party.'

Once he had rid himself of the bad wine, he was remarkably restored and cheerfully set himself to sleep after the attendant and I had cleaned him up. As for me, I knew I had to get up and out of the place. I wanted to lie down and I wanted fresh air.

'Just lend me a couple of blankets,' I told the attendant and I took myself off. I had noticed earlier the lifeboats slung up over the decks. There was no overcrowding in there. I climbed in amongst the rescue kit and iron rations, wrapped myself in blankets and went to sleep for what was left of the night under a swinging sky.

There was some consternation when I emerged in daylight amongst a squad of men scrubbing down the decks but I was ready to deal with anyone who might complain, and nobody did. Scant attention had been paid to the Q.A.s on board until our help was needed. I felt that somebody, somewhere should have said thank-you. My patient was up and dressed when I reached the Sick Bay and walked ashore with the rest of us when we landed at Dover.

Britain was full of activity. The defences of an island at war were being energetically removed, anti-tank traps and road blocks demolished, barbed wire defences rolled away. House-wives gleefully pulled down the black-out curtains and rueful car-owners looked over their vehicles which had spent 'the duration' on blocks in the garage. Demobilised men and women were looking anxiously for jobs. Pat Fuller's demobilisation date was 12th November. He would sail from India in October.

In the second week of September, at the end of my leave, I returned to Europe. The 86th with Pat Kavanagh and Pin with her hospital were even then on the way to India. My old unit, 75th B.G.H. was in Norway, helping with civil administration there after the chaos of German occupation. I joined the 105th B.G.H. at De Haan in Belgium and was put in charge of a ward of German officers suffering from dysentery as a result of insanitary conditions in their P.O.W. camp. The responsible administrator was given a 'bowler hat' for his negligence. I made use of this new nursing experience by increasing my German vocabulary, even though the field was somewhat specialised and unsocial. It must have amused the German officers whose barrack-room phrases I was studiously learning, for I was otherwise strictly professional towards them.

'Sister!' said the new M.O. in horror. 'Where did you pick up that language?' He had read modern languages before taking up medicine.

De Haan had been a popular seaside resort in peacetime and now, with its shore checked daily for tidal mines, it provided a perfect playground for members of the Forces stationed in the area. We lay on the beach in the last of the September sun and used the German pillboxes as changing rooms for swimming.

On 11th November the *Athlone Castle*, bearing ex-prisoners of war from Japanese camps and 'demob.' soldiers which included Pat Fuller, docked in Southampton. The P.O.W.s were the first to leave the ship. Bands played and crowds cheered as these fortunate survivors set foot on English soil once more. The demob. soldiers followed and were instructed to report to specific centres a few days later. At one of these, Major Fuller, now Mr. Fuller, was given a cardboard box containing a suit of his own choosing, a pair of shoes, a raincoat and a trilby hat, six shillings travel allowance and ten weeks' supply of tobacco.

'I hope you'll still love me without the uniform,' he wrote, suddenly doubtful. He would have to wait for my next leave, due in December, to find out.

When it came, he met me in Victoria Station and any doubts were dispelled. I knew that I had made the right decision in not going to India. On Christmas Day we became engaged and on 2nd January 1946 I returned to De Haan to find that the 105th B.G.H. was disbanding. Perhaps, with luck, I would get a United Kingdom posting? But no, I went back into Germany, to join the 77th B.H.G. at Wuppertal, an industrial centre of little attraction. Pat was left to pick up his career in shipping at the point where he had left it six years previously and to hunt about in ravaged Britain for somewhere for us to live.

The War Office was losing patience with me. My next request, for a compassionate posting to Britain in order to be married was ignored. The winter passed in Wuppertal and little German boys with toboggans skimmed down the snowy slopes dexterously avoiding wrecked tanks and guns. Our April wedding had to be postoned and Pat's letters were becoming increasingly anxious as he juggled with church banns, relatives and estate agents.

'People are beginning to think you are a figment of my imagination,' he complained.

Not till March did my posting come and I left the British Army of the Rhine (B.A.O.R.) for the last time. Our wedding day was fixed for the second anniversary of D-Day, 6th June 1946. Until that date, I was to nurse soldiers suffering from tuberculosis in Shaftesbury Military Hospital.

Tuberculosis was still a killer at that time and the long, airy ward I took over contained thirty-six men whose lungs were affected, some very badly, by the disease. In some cases, the poor living conditions of prisoner-of-war camps were responsible. Other men, Commando-trained to live and fight in any circumstances, had tried their physical resources too far, like the sergeant who had been a member of a special mission air-drop over Jugoslavia. He had lived for weeks in a damp cave without dry clothing or nourishing food and now his once superb physique was a shell around hopelessly infected lungs. With others, there seemed to be no explanation for the tell-tale shadow on the X-Ray plate. Such a one was Corporal Baines, who, carrying his kitbag on his shoulder off the ship from India on his way to demobilisation, walked confidently through the compulsory chest X-Ray screening, and was stunned to find he had a patch on one lung. No more carrying kitbags for him, no long-awaited reunion with his girl, but a bed in Shaftesbury Hospital and a programme of rest, blood tests, sputum tests and X-Rays.

I was under no special risk in the T.B. ward as my blood showed that I had plenty of active antibodies, which was something to do with that scar on my neck which had so offended Tommy Gibson. The gland removed when I was a child was probably tubercular.

Rest was the key word of the treatment here. This was before the days of drug therapy and hopes were pinned on rest, good food and fresh air with supportive medicines. When that failed, surgery was used to collapse and therefore rest the damaged lung. Sections of rib sometimes had to be removed in order to release painful adhesions. The final surgery was removal of the lung. Prognosis was not good yet when I met my new patients, it was hard to believe they were so diseased. Sergeant Headingly for instance, was up and about, with his stripes sewn on his dressing-gown sleeve, his face ruddy with health, it seemed. He collected tit-bits for the weekly ward magazine he edited. His X-Ray plates showed the other side of the story. The handful of men who would never leave their beds again had dry, racking coughs that made one's own chest ache to hear.

Psychologically, it was a difficult ward to handle, since most of the men felt fairly well for most of the time and rebelled against enforced rest. On their good days, they wanted to go home, to start work, anything but the boredom of quietly rest-ing until blood and sputum were free from tubercle. And when, week after week, X-Rays showed no improvement, terrible but understandable depression gripped even the most balanced of men. None of the treatments which we relied upon at that time produced dramatic changes. Recovery was slow and sometimes temporary. Our M.O. was patient in the extreme, tactfully forgetting things said in anger and holding out hope and encouragement all the time. I had an excellent V.A.D. nurse to help me, a cheerful girl full of bright ideas to keep the men's minds occupied. From time to time, we contributed to the ward 'Rag'.

There were the good moments when real improvement was seen and a man was judged well enough to go home on the condition that he reported back to the hospital at intervals. There were the bad times when, little by little, in the case of a man whose lungs were not responding, activities would be curtailed. Breakfast would be served in bed in the future and there would be no more trips to the hospital shop, up only for toilet and later, not even that. With the loss of a man's occupa-tion went his self-confidence. Blood in his sputum would be next. Doctors were still fumbling for the answer to tuberculosis.

I became very attached to all the ward and was very touched by a little ceremony in my honour when the time came for me to leave. In the centre of the ward one day, after a few words from the M.O., my V.A.D. presented me with an elegant table lamp, my wedding present from them all.

It was rest period. The men lay on their beds the length of the ward, each face turned towards me, smiling at my embarrassment. I was at a loss to know how to thank them and reverted to childhood, planting a kiss on each forehead. It was not at all professional. Nurses do not kiss their patients, but it seemed the right thing for me to do.

'Now the M.O.!' changed the men delightedly, and the curtain came down on my grand finale. Q.A. P/294203 was no more.

With general demobilisation of all the Forces, thousands of faces began the long, gradual process of being forgotten. The Private Eastons went back to the farms to relieve the girls of the Land Army. The Duncans went back to postal delivery and men like Boney returned to the classroom. My Q.A. friends scattered in an explosion of marriages or new careers that took them to the four corners of the earth; Soutie to Malaya, Duff to South America, Joan Deadman to Canada, Annie P. Scott to Baghdad, 'Andy' and myself to Australia.

'She'll no' persuade me to live in that nasty hot place.' Andy's life-long friend, Janet, stayed behind to become a Matron in Scotland.

Now, so many years later, most of us are back in England. Some are comfortable grandmothers. Each moves in a different circle but when we meet, as we regularly do, the common memory of a huge experience holds us together. We do not dwell on the war years. We have no constant reminder as so many of the men we nursed must surely suffer. My friends and I have two legs each and two arms. We are not blind. Our noses are our own. Yet I am left with the eternal question of what happened to those brave jokers who were so grossly mutilated that to have given their lives would have been no greater sacrifice. Each time I see a man with obvious signs of plastic surgery or disablement, I rapidly calculate his age. Could he have been one of my wounded heroes?

And Selzinski and all the other victims of the concentration camps, what became of them? The questions keep coming.

On an overnight trip from Toronto to Boston in 1973, I met a Polish woman. She spoke very little English and when we were requested to change coaches at Buffalo she demanded of the driver in a rough sort of German if we had already reached Boston. Her sister in Canada had put her on the coach with instructions to stay there until it stopped, which would be in Boston. Neither the driver nor any of the American travellers returning from holiday in Canada, laden with presents and sleepy children, could understand a word she said as, still wildly questioning, she was nudged down the bus steps and into the station waiting-room.

I went over to her. 'Stay by me,' I said. 'I too am going to Boston.'

Her joy at finding someone who understood her was over-whelming and she rewarded me with an account of herself which lasted through most of the night and kept all of us in the coach awake. The curious slang she used was very familiar to me. It was the German of the concentration camps.

'Look, I'm a sick woman,' she said and opened her big black handbag to show me her collection of pill bottles. 'I got blood pressure and my heart is no good. I was six years in a German concentration camp.'

The woman across the aisle shushed us and said didn't we know that some folk wanted to sleep.

'I got bladder trouble and only one good kidney.' My companion swallowed a couple of pills at a gulp. 'And look at this.' She pulled up he sleeve and, in the flitting lights from Neon signs as we sped past 'All Nite Hamburger' joints, I saw a long, puckered scar. 'Injections,' she said in a throaty whisper. 'Experimenting with us women.'

She had come to live with her sister in Canada who had wisely fled from Poland in 1938 but in reality, my companion had never left the camp. Are they all like this?

She was met the next morning in Boston by ner nephew, a straight-up-and-down American soldier who took her away, happily disregarding all his auntie's querulous complaints. She hurried to keep up with him on legs heavy with oedema and clutching her bag of pills.

Today, my grandchildren play on the lawn outside my window. There is a small boy in a moth-eaten Q.A. battle-dress jacket and a German tin hat. They have been in the dress-up box again.

'Bang! Bang! You're dead.' Everyone had a different war. This was mine.

Index